WALKING *Lois* HOME

WALKING *Lois* HOME

LIVING OUT OUR CHRISTIAN CALL TO LOVE THE SICK AND DYING

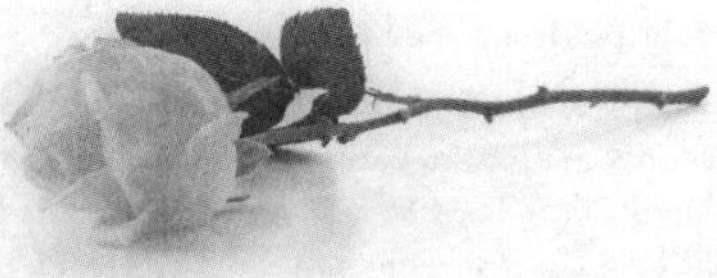

Michael and Tracy Balboni

BakerBooks
a division of Baker Publishing Group
Grand Rapids, Michigan

Published by Baker Books
a division of Baker Publishing Group
Grand Rapids, Michigan
BakerBooks.com

Printed in the United States of America

Library of Congress Cataloging-in-Publication Data
Names: Balboni, Michael J. author | Balboni, Tracy A. author
Title: Walking Lois home : living out our Christian call to love the sick and dying / Michael and Tracy Balboni.
Description: Grand Rapids, Michigan : Baker Books, a division of Baker Publishing Group, [2026]
Identifiers: LCCN 2026007725 | ISBN 9781540905437 paperback | ISBN 9781493456529 ebook
Subjects: LCSH: Healing—Religious aspects—Christianity | Caregivers——Religious life | Grief—Religious aspects—Christianity | Bereavement—Religious aspects—Christianity
Classification: LCC BT732 .B3375 2026
LC record available at https://lccn.loc.gov/2026007725

Cover design by Sarah Gordon

Published in association with Books & Such Literary Management www.booksandsuch.com.

Baker Publishing Group publications use paper produced from sustainable forestry practices and postconsumer waste whenever possible.

26 27 28 29 30 31 32 7 6 5 4 3 2 1

Tracy and Michael dedicate this book to their dear friend
Lois Ann Meinhardt

Tracy dedicates this book to her parents,
each of whom has taught her the art of caring for the sick:
Dr. Elizabeth M. Spencer-Smith
Dr. Barry A. Smith
Dr. Richard M. Timms

She also dedicates this book to
Restoration Fellowship in Boston,
a church home that has brought new life,
joy, and healing in Christ

Michael dedicates this book to his parents,
who have been his greatest examples
of faithfulness, hospitality, and sacrifice:
Benedetta Balboni
Edmund S. Balboni

He also dedicates this book to Park Street Church,
where he learned the joys and challenges of pastoring,
and where many stepped forward in loving care of Lois

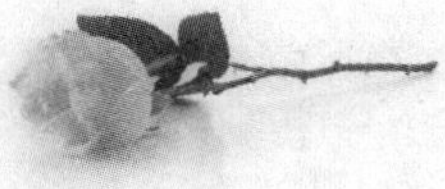

Contents

Part 3 Walking the Path Together

Note to the Reader

All names and identifying information in this book, unless explicitly permitted, has been changed to protect the confidentiality and anonymity of individuals and institutions discussed. While certain details have been altered, the stories and the essence of each conversation accurately reflect our lived experiences, individually as a physician and a pastor, and collectively as a couple.

The telling of the story of Lois Meinhardt is with her express permission and encouragement. The writing of this book was, in fact, Lois's idea that she raised while she received care in our home. Her story is told from our perspectives as best we can remember the details, some of which were recorded in our private journals and others based on our collective memory. We have attempted to accurately reflect Lois's story as we experienced it, though—as in any telling of the past—there may be imperfections in details. Many others cared for Lois alongside us, and some details of Lois's life were obtained from conversations with those persons.

The stories of others described in this book—Arthur, Joy, Pastor David, Richard, Dr. Patel, Dawn, Helen, Mike, Margaret, Irene, Pastor Brian, Nurse Patrick, Peter, Kevin, Sharon, Dr. Kearney, Chaplain Betsy, and Mary—are based on real persons. These individuals are people we cared for directly or those we interviewed about their experiences. In all cases, names and other identifying details have been changed to maintain confidentiality.

All quotes from clergy are drawn from our National Clergy Study on End-of-Life Care, which was funded by the National Cancer Institute. This study was completed in 2015 and included a national survey of randomly selected clergy around the United States. We also conducted one-on-one, audio-recorded interviews and focus groups of clergy from Massachusetts, Illinois, Texas, and California. The quotes are drawn from our prior publications and the underlying database.

AI was used to assist with grammar, occasional flow, and clarity. The book's structure, stories, content, and writing are our own, unless otherwise noted.

Part 1

Losing Our Way in Death Denial

One

Introduction

For my dear broken people, I'm heartbroken.
  I weep, seized by grief.
Are there no healing ointments in Gilead?
  Isn't there a doctor in the house?
So why can't something be done
  to heal and save my dear, dear people?

Jeremiah 8:21–22 MSG

Broken by Bad News

Lois held her breath. Her right hand covered her mouth in shock, pulling her blue mask down off her nose. She closed her brown eyes tightly. Silence passed, and the young doctor, whom Lois thought looked no older than a teenager, shifted uncomfortably in his chair before speaking again, his expression hidden under the large mask covering all but his eyes.

"I'm sorry, Ms. Meinhardt, to have to give you this bad news. We will need to do surgery to remove the tumor. This will mean you'll lose that kidney, but you should do just fine with one. We'll probably be able to get you onto my OR schedule in about three weeks."

Lois's hand had fallen back to her side as Dr. Lee was speaking. Her mask was now pulled down below her chin awkwardly. She took shallow breaths, gripping the edges of her chair tightly, feeling as if she were going to fall to the ground. Dr. Lee kept talking, his words muffled through his mask, but Lois heard none of what was said. She was alone, entirely alone. She eventually let go of the chair and bowed her head into both hands.

"I can't do this," she said softly, shaking her head. "I just can't do this."

Dr. Lee stopped speaking as Lois's words interrupted his rehearsal of the risks and benefits of surgery. There was silence again. Lois's face remained hidden in her hands. He stood up abruptly, glancing at his watch.

"Ms. Meinhardt, I'm going to step out and get Jenny, the nurse I work with. She can help you think through the procedure, and she can also get you in touch with one of our social workers if you need additional help."

He walked out the door. Lois's body jerked at the sound of it clanging shut behind him.

The remainder of the appointment was a blur. Lois spoke to Jenny and signed some forms. She didn't bother reading them and had quickly stuffed copies into her large pocketbook. She was in her car now, a fading blue 2003 Pontiac Grand Prix, driving slowly back to her apartment in a subsidized elder housing unit in Winthrop, Massachusetts. A light drizzle kept her windshield wipers beating slowly over the glass. The late-April day was gray and cold, and Lois shivered despite the thick navy wool skirt suit she wore, which pulled uncomfortably over her plump, seventy-three-year-old waist and hips. Her fake-pearl necklace and clip-on earrings, accessories she'd added so meticulously that morning as she readied herself for her appointment, now felt cold and heavy.

She pulled the earrings off at the next stoplight, leaving them in the console between the two front seats.

Suddenly, as she stared at two people hurrying across the intersection, carrying umbrellas that waved in the gusts of wind, a jarring thought entered her mind.

I could kill myself.

She was confused by the flood of emotions that attended this thought, which included both fear and elation. She felt terrified of death and wondered how in the world she could do it. What if it was painful? And yet, she was also elated. Death could be her escape. Alone, with no money, no family, and few friends, now she was facing cancer. Her younger self could never have imagined being in such a place. She had to escape.

The person in the car behind her laid on his horn, annoyed. The light had turned green. Lois was still lost in a landslide of emotions. She shook her head and stepped abruptly on the gas, causing the car to jerk into the intersection. She continued slowly down the road leading to her apartment building. The man in the car behind her drove into the oncoming lane to pass her, pausing as his passenger window came abreast with hers. He yelled something at her she couldn't hear. Lois looked vacantly into his angry face. He accelerated and raced on ahead.

Lois parked in the same spot she always did, letting the engine sputter to a halt. She remained in the driver's seat, unmoving. Peering through her windshield covered in streams of silvery raindrops, she saw beyond the nearly vacant parking lot to the ocean. A lone fishing boat was moving slowly by. She followed it with her eyes until it disappeared behind the dull 1960s square architecture of her apartment building. Now the ocean water blended imperceptibly with the clouds—an empty, endless gray mist.

The stillness captured her, drawing her back into memories of her childhood and being at the beach with her parents. They had been poor, but she hadn't known that until her teens. Lois was a child who'd arrived after years of infertility to parents in their late forties, and they adored her—particularly her father. She remembered Sundays after church, playing on the beach while her parents strolled together.

Going to church had been their Sunday morning ritual when she was a girl. Her parents loved church. Lois hadn't thought of church much since childhood, until about a year ago. Loneliness had crept up on her when her work as an art teacher at various Boston elementary schools came to an end. She had been laid off at age sixty-nine, and for a few years she did some substitute teaching. But then the calls stopped coming. She tried to fill her time and supplement her meager social security income by doing ballroom dancing lessons and performances. Then one morning in June 2019, after a lonely Saturday evening, Lois headed back to her childhood sanctuary for the 11:00 a.m. service. She carefully dressed in her dark flowered dress with a matching cardigan and her fake pearls. She sat where she had with her parents so many decades prior, in the middle set of pews toward the back. As she listened to the organ, to the choir, she closed her eyes.

After the service, Lois went out to the Boston Common across from the church for a lunch being held there. She felt anxious, knowing nobody. One of the ministers, noticing that she looked lost, approached her and shook her hand. "Hello, I'm Pastor Michael. What's your name?"

Lois talked with him for some time, even sharing with him about her loneliness. "I'm a bit surprised to be telling you this!" she admitted.

"It's okay. You're hardly the only one. I'm just so glad you came today."

Explaining that he would like to help connect Lois with the church community, Pastor Michael gave her his cell phone number, writing it on the side of the church program she was holding. She received it gratefully and said that she would call later that week, even as doubts filled her head. *He's just being nice. He's too busy. I'll figure this out on my own.*

That had been ten months ago. Now her eyes moved from her gaze toward the ocean to her purse in the seat beside her. She pulled out the medical forms and found her date book, tightly wrapped with several rubber bands to keep various papers tucked inside the front cover from falling out. She took off the bands and fumbled through the papers. And there it was: the folded and worn church program dated June 16, 2019, with the handwritten phone number on the side. She pulled out her flip phone, hesitated a moment, and then her trembling fingers began dialing. The phone rang once, twice, then three times. Lois's heart sank. But then the fourth ring was cut short.

"Hello, this is Pastor Michael."

Lois took a deep breath. Finally, she spoke in her strong Boston accent. "Hello, Pastor. My name is Lois Meinhardt. We met last summer at your church picnic. I . . . I am calling because . . ." There was a long pause. "I'm calling because I . . . " Her voice was high-pitched and halting, trailing off as she couldn't find further words. Lois then began to sob.

This is when we, Michael and Tracy, began a journey with Lois. Along with many others from our church community, we would walk with Lois through serious illness, all the way home.

Rediscovering Care of the Sick

Matthew 25:37–40 says, "'Master, what are you talking about? When did we ever see you hungry and feed you, thirsty and give you a drink? And when did we ever see you sick or in prison and come to you?' Then the King will say, 'I'm telling the solemn truth: Whenever you did one of these things to someone overlooked or ignored, that was me—you did it to me'" (MSG).

Caring for the sick is a fundamental spiritual practice for Christians. When Jesus performed powerful, healing miracles, he did so as a sign that his kingdom—the kingdom of God—had arrived. Then Jesus empowered his disciples to do the same: "Jesus called his twelve disciples to him and gave them authority to drive out impure spirits and to heal every disease and sickness" (Matt. 10:1 NIV).

Responding to Jesus's calling, Christians have cared for the sick as a sign that Jesus remains King and Healer. Church history is replete with examples. Early Christians attended to persons suffering from the plague.[1] Looking to God's heavenly kingdom, Christians risked and at times contracted deadly diseases from those under their care. In the third century, Bishop Dionysius of Alexandria described the commonplace poor treatment of the ill during the plague and its sharp contrast to the response of Christians:

> At the first onset of disease, they pushed the sufferers away and fled from their dearest, throwing them into the roads before they were dead and treating unburied corpses as dirt. . . . [By contrast] most of our brother Christians showed unbounded love and loyalty, never sparing themselves and thinking only of one another. Heedless of danger, they took charge of the sick, attending to their every need and ministering to them in Christ.[2]

Among the Greeks and Romans, the responsibility to take care of the sick fell fully on family members.[3] With the exception of well-paid physicians, strangers were not involved. When people fell ill, it was common to believe that the illness was divine punishment. The sick were considered judged and in that sense responsible for their illness. Jesus's vision of the sick led Christians to reject Greco-Roman beliefs about illness. Illness was not a punishment. Rather, God was believed to be present in suffering. In contrast to being cursed, to suffer illness meant to be uniquely joined with Christ, the Ultimate Sufferer (Matt. 25:40).[4] Likewise, care for the sick was not exclusively a family responsibility. Jesus taught about the good Samaritan who poured "oil and wine" on a nearly dead stranger. The effort and cost of providing care to the sick were responsibilities of Christians, motivated by love of neighbor, regardless of whether the ill person was family or a stranger (Luke 10:29–37).

Boldly caring for plague victims in the early centuries after Jesus's death and resurrection was only the beginning. Christians throughout history have demonstrated a recognition of Jesus's call to show hospitality to the sick. In the fourth century, Basil the Bishop of Caesarea began the first hospital, located in modern-day Turkey. The three-hundred-bed facility included a hospice and a dedicated ward for those with leprosy.[5] This was the first of many hospitals built by Christians, from ancient times to the present day. Even the term *hospital* echoes Jesus's call to care for the sick. The Latin root *hosti* means the embrace of stranger as guest—or love of stranger.[6] In the New Testament, the Greek word for hospitality is *philoxenia*, or "love of stranger." During the Middle Ages, Benedictine monks bowed before the sick person arriving at the monastery for their care, poignantly displaying their love for the sick person as Christ himself. In the 1800s, Florence Nightingale, responding to a call from God to care for the sick, revolutionized care for wounded soldiers and spearheaded the development of the nursing profession. And in the twentieth century, Dame Cicely Saunders, responding to a "tapping on the shoulder" from God, dedicated her work as a physician to improve care for the dying, ultimately inaugurating the hospice movement.[7] Jesus's kingdom vision of care for the sick as if they were Jesus himself has shaped medicine's history as well as its practice today.

How does the contemporary church answer Jesus's call to care for the sick? Though the response has continued in an unbroken stream since early Christians' hazardous embrace of plague victims, it is a trickle now in comparison. Is the church willing to take the same bold risks today? Do those opportunities even exist?

Of course, many areas of the world remain without, or with only rudimentary, medical infrastructure, and the church does indeed have a long and needed calling to provide medical care in those settings—also known as Christian medical missions. Christian medical missions will continue to have a critical role in fulfilling the call to care for the sick. But is that the only setting for us to boldly respond to Christ's appeal to *all* of his disciples to "heal every disease and sickness" (Matt. 10:1 NIV)?

As Western medicine has grown in complexity and specialization, it has increasingly dominated the care of the sick. The highly advanced medical systems in most modern societies make it appear that Christians no longer need to step in to care for those who are unwell. Reflecting this shift, most hospitals with Christian origins have lost their core Christian spiritual identities, caring only for the physical body without consideration of the person's inner needs. As scientific medicine has grown, Christians have largely lost the centrality of Jesus's call to care for the sick, both body and soul.

Understanding and Responding in Three Parts

When we first met Lois, we saw up close the gap between the church's calling to care for the sick and how that care often unfolds in real life. This book is a byproduct of that reality, pointing toward a way the church can recover Jesus's call and be empowered to walk with people who are seriously ill.[8] In a world where physical care depends heavily on institutions and technology, the church is invited to reclaim its role in healing. How can the church better bridge the distance between high-tech medicine, which can feel deeply impersonal, and the call to love the sick and shepherd them all the way home? When ill persons, like Lois, cry out for help, how should the church respond?

This book follows our journey with Lois Meinhardt, a woman we did not know when she reached out in desperation in April

2020. Newly diagnosed with kidney cancer, Lois was overwhelmed and at times suicidal. Michael entered her story first, walking with her as a pastor, listening, praying, and gathering church members to offer practical help. After surgery in June 2020 to remove her cancerous kidney, Lois returned home hoping the worst was over. Instead, by October 2020, scans revealed the cancer had spread to her bones and lungs. Her care included repeated encounters with a strained medical system, including for chemotherapy, multiple surgeries, hospitalizations, and a long skilled nursing facility stay.

As her illness advanced, Lois asked if Tracy could be involved as a medical adviser while remaining outside her formal care team. Tracy's role as a physician allowed her to be present in hospital rooms during COVID when others could not, offering her advocacy and steady presence. In January 2021, after another hospitalization for a cancer-related arm fracture, Lois faced a choice between more treatment and hospice care. She entered inpatient hospice, but it soon became clear she would not be allowed to remain there and would be sent to a facility where visitors were highly restricted. During those weeks, we both came to the same conviction that Lois should not die alone. In early February 2021, Lois came to live in our home under hospice care, where she spent the final six months of her life.

The chapters that follow trace our shared journey with Lois, not only as a medical story but also as a human and spiritual one. Several chapters introduce others we have known or cared for in our roles as physician or pastor. Each story is unique, yet together they offer a shared witness from which we can learn and grow. If you are facing serious illness or caring for someone with illness, our prayer is that these reflections will be used by God's Spirit to provide wisdom, guidance, and hope for the journey. If you are reflecting on the church community's call to love the sick and dying, we pray the Holy Spirit will work through these reflections to illuminate and energize that calling. We invite you to journey with us through three parts of this book.

Part 1 explores the cultural shifts that have shaped the church's loss of vision for caring for the sick. This includes a weakened Christian understanding of the relationship between spirituality and health, alongside the growing influence of a materialistic approach within modern medicine. These chapters show how this loss of vision has often left the sick unseen or forgotten and point toward the need for a renewed theology of Christian care.

Part 2 offers a Christian theology of health, illness, and death to guide ill persons and their caretakers in modern medical settings. Christians sometimes emphasize certain beliefs, such as God's power to heal, while overlooking other essential teachings, such as preparing faithfully for death, addressing fears, or knowing when to let go. When illness comes, this imbalance can lead to confusion or even harm. To address this, each chapter centers on one of the last seven sayings of Christ on the cross, drawing wisdom for the spiritual struggles and questions that arise in serious illness.

Part 3 turns to the calling of the body of Christ to respond together to suffering. When one person becomes sick, the whole church is affected. The Spirit forms the church as a community of love called to respond to the sick. The church is to be a community of action, offering practical help and support. It is to be a community of presence, staying close, listening carefully, and showing up even when there are no words. And it is to be a community of faith, holding fast to the promises of resurrection and eternal life. As a community of action, presence, and belief, the church becomes a living witness of Christ's love for the sick, the dying, and those who grieve.

A Marriage of Two Worlds

We will explore these issues by bringing together Christian theology, scientific research, and real experiences of illness.[9] Theological reflection and the scientific study of an ordered universe complement one another as two lenses that clarify our vision. When held side by side, they bring into focus a renewed Christian approach to caring for the sick.

We have had the joy and challenge of working together at the intersection of serious illness, medicine, theology, and the church for the past twenty-five years. As a physician and a pastor, we have often understood our own marriage to be a living symbol of what many assume cannot fit together. In us, the world of medical science on the one hand, and the world of theology and the church on the other hand, have found a home together. Our life together has shown us that these two realms, which are often separated or placed in tension, can live in harmony, even a joyful union. During these years, we have been called to study, teach, and practice how faith and medicine shape and strengthen one another.

Our first book, *Hostility to Hospitality*, has been described as a prophetic word to the secular academic medical community.[10] It warns about the dangers of a spirituality of immanence: a way of thinking that values only what is material, measurable, and useful. We argue that this mindset has been slowly consuming the best parts of medicine and the institutions that support it. That book calls upon secular medicine to reconsider its unnecessary and destructive divorce from religion and spirituality.

Our hope is that this new book—as enabled by God—might become a prophetic word to the church. We believe that this same spirituality of immanence has been shaping how Christians think about sickness and health. It has created a false division between medicine and the church, leading many believers to approach illness with distorted theology and little understanding of how to live faithfully within sickness or how to care well for those who are ill. As a result, the church's long and rich calling to love the sick in Jesus's name has been weakened.

Lois pleaded with us to write this book as a way of telling her story and helping others and the church learn how to journey through the dangerous landscape of illness. Our experience of caring for Lois during the final year of her life made this need even more real for us. We experienced in Lois how ill persons have their own unique calling to the Christian community. As our community cared for her broken body, we witnessed up close the inevitable losses of earthly hopes; and as her hope turned to God in a remarkable spiritual transformation, she embodied to us the beautiful reality of our hope in Jesus for the eternal life to come. Walking with her through serious illness and eventually bringing her into our own home so she could die surrounded by love showed us that the care of the sick cannot be limited to professional roles alone. It requires sacrifice and must be shared by the entire faith community. Such shared care is not only an act of compassion but also a powerful living witness of Christ's love. This was once central to Christian community life. We believe this call must be reclaimed.

Two

It

> Ivan Ilych saw that he was dying, and he was in continual despair. . . . He simply did not and could not grasp it. . . . [He] would turn his attention to it and try to drive the thought of it away, but without success. It would come and stand before him and look at him, and he would be petrified, and the light would die out of his eyes, and he would again begin asking himself whether IT alone was true.
>
> Leo Tolstoy

> The waning days of our lives are given over to treatments that addle our brains and sap our bodies for a sliver's chance of benefit. . . . Lacking a coherent view of how people might live successfully all the way to their very end, we have allowed our fates to be controlled by the imperatives of medicine, technology, and strangers.
>
> Atul Gawande

AT THE SAME TIME Lois was beginning her journey through cancer, Arthur's course came to an abrupt end as he succumbed to what Tolstoy referred to as simply *It*. The inevitability of death.

Arthur's trek began seven years prior. One morning after a bowel movement, he found the toilet filled with blood—*his blood.* He had ignored the dots of dark red in the toilet water over the prior months. Now the stark contrast of the bright red blood against the white porcelain couldn't be ignored. His throat tightened with anxiety.

Five days later, Arthur lay on a gurney after his colonoscopy. The doctor walked away after a brief conversation with Arthur and his wife, Joy, about the test results. Arthur looked at his wife through a blur of tears. "I got *It*. I have colon cancer."

Joy gripped his hand with both of hers. "So what? We are with God. He is with us. We will fight *It*. We'll take care of *It*. We are in this together."

Fight *It* they did. Joy and Arthur went to the most highly acclaimed doctors in Boston, New York, and Rochester. They pursued alternative therapies from extreme juicing to chiropractic remedies. They expended large sums of money to travel to South America to receive care from healers touting cures to even the most aggressive cancers. Their church community prayed. Their pastor, David, visited and prayed with fervency for healing.

Arthur desperately wanted to live. Joy believed anything was possible with God.

Arthur loved life. He loved people, especially his family. He would regularly host lavish meals and spend long hours conversing and laughing with family and friends over drinks. His vivacity and charisma led to him and Joy living the American dream. The son of poor immigrants, he was a self-made, successful businessman with many friends. Joy lovingly described him as "the guy who could get anything done . . . because he was so relational."

With the same passion and determination that characterized his life up to his cancer diagnosis, Arthur pursued his quest to defeat *It*. But after seven years of ultimately unsuccessful surgeries, radiation therapy, chemotherapies, and clinical trials, his spirit altered. Joy solemnly recalled the transformation of her husband. "Something went hugely wrong. . . . Arthur lost being Arthur. He turned inward. His soul turned dark."

"My heart aches for him," Joy admitted, "because God granted our prayer for longer life but he was miserable."

Rather than living well, Arthur was dodging *It*. And as *It* relentlessly pursued him, he became increasingly gripped by unspoken fear. Joy described how he "pulled me and his kids into his fear, like a black hole." Most nights he could only fitfully sleep. Joy would regularly awaken to Arthur pacing the floor, incoherently mumbling.

Near the end of his life, Arthur shared with his wife the conversation he had with his psychologist in what would be his last counseling appointment. He said to Joy, "I told her that I think there is a demon inside me. *It* won't let me go. I can't sit. I can't sleep. I don't want to be alone. I'm leaving a mess of my marriage. It's not going to be good for the family when I leave." Joy responded with consoling words, but his dark mood remained unaltered.

Arthur had a special connection with Pastor David. His visits would include friendly conversation as well as prayers for healing and peace over Arthur. David reflected on the close connection they enjoyed in those visits stemming from "a complete convergence between my prayers for healing, the emotional connection and camaraderie we had between us, and the physical healing Arthur so deeply wanted."

But David also suspected that Arthur's time was short. And so he found an opportunity to raise the issue of Arthur's preparation for death. During a lull in their conversation, he broached the topic with pointed questions.

"Arthur, maybe the time has come for us to talk about being ready to meet our Maker? Do you have peace?"

Without hesitation, Arthur shot back, "I don't want to think about that. To think that way is to give up. I want to fight this.

That's what we should do. So no, I don't want to talk about making peace." Arthur's eyes closed, and he was silent.

David, understanding that he was now dismissed, gently replied, "Arthur, thank you for your time. I love you, and I will be praying for your healing."

Without opening his eyes, Arthur tersely responded, "Thank you."

These were their last words. Within a few days, Arthur fell into unconsciousness and died.

From Tame to Taboo

Like Arthur, or Tolstoy's fictional character Ivan Ilyich, we often resist facing our mortality, even when death is undeniably imminent.

Clinicians often struggle to communicate to their patients the realities of dying. In one study of patients with advanced cancer, Mack and colleagues found that end-of-life discussions often happened late in the illness, usually during hospital stays and sometimes with doctors other than the patient's primary oncologist.[1] In a systematic review of communication in palliative care, researchers found that doctors struggle with these conversations because they find them emotionally difficult, they worry about taking away hope, they are unsure about the prognosis, and they often lack time.[2] Together, these studies show that physicians frequently have these conversations later than needed and face several barriers that make them difficult to initiate.

While clinicians struggle to speak with patients about dying, many patients also don't want to hear it. In one study, 86 percent of those with a fatal lung disease did not want to talk about the end of life but would "rather concentrate on staying alive than talk about death."[3] Another study reported that among nine thousand terminally ill patients, less than half were aware of their terminal diagnosis.[4]

Denial of death has not always been so common. From the early church through the Middle Ages, as Lydia Dugdale explains, Christian communities expected and accepted illness and death as a necessary step from a limited and broken world into a perfect and eternal heaven.[5] This understanding cultivated a simplicity in Christians' approach to death. Solzhenitsyn writes, "They took death calmly . . . and they departed easily, as if they were just moving into a new house."[6] Historian Philippe Ariès describes this older viewpoint of death as "tame."[7] Rather than being viewed as "wild" or out of control, death was accepted with trust because it was not the end but a new beginning. This tame view of death reduced fear and encouraged hope for the continuation of life after death.

The "tame" understanding of death also allowed agency, purpose, and meaning for dying persons. The dying had important tasks to accomplish that were solely in their control. The dying person found meaning and purpose in their own anticipation and planning for the eternal life to come following death. They had agency or could take control of their dying through practices that cultivated preparation, such as those found in the *Ars moriendi*.[8] Translated from Latin as "The Art of Dying," these guidebooks offer illustrations and teachings on how to die well according to biblical beliefs. Written soon after the Black Plague in 1415 and 1450, they were widely popular and were translated into most Western European languages.

A "tame" death was also close in proximity to the living. Most people died at home. Corpses remained there for days, allowing for visitation and lament among family and friends. Visitation of the person after death provided an embodied symbol of the reality of the loved one's eternal presence beyond death. Burial was a literal act of placing the body, like a seed, into the ground to await the promised resurrection (John 12:24; 1 Cor. 15:42–48). Graveyards were close to town centers and churches, enabling ongoing visits to gravesites, themselves tangible reminders of the eternal presence of departed loved ones. As an anticipated end result of the sinfulness of the world, death brought deep sadness. Yet, for Christians, death also was imbued with a hope far greater than any found in this world—the hope of eternal life.

In the early years of the twentieth century, this "tame" death was replaced by a "wild" death so dreadful it was best denied. Death became taboo. According to Ariès, death became a shameful topic to meditate on or openly discuss. Now even the seriously ill, like Arthur, find death too "wild" to hold in one's thoughts.

What has made death taboo? Significant changes in society have made it increasingly hidden and unfamiliar. Alongside these shifts, hope has moved from being rooted in the promise of eternal life to being centered on the present world, even among many Christians. We'll consider first the social shifts that have increasingly rendered death more deniable.

Public health and other social programs. One result of better public health and social welfare programs is that we live longer, healthier lives. Average life expectancy in 1900 was forty-seven years old. By the year 2000, it had increased to seventy-seven years old. Social flourishing, longer lives, and fewer deaths create a psychology of human security.[9] Denying death becomes more justifiable because life feels secure.

Location of death. Before the twentieth century, most people died at home. The reality of death was softened by occurring in the family context because dying was familiar to all. With the rise of hospitals during the twentieth century, including through government support for health care, the place of death shifted from the home to hospitals. Deaths in a hospital went from less than 5 percent of deaths in the US in 1900, to 33 percent in 1940, and to 78 percent by the early 1990s. As of 2017, in the US approximately 70 percent of individuals die in a hospital or nursing facility.[10] Though most people prefer to die at home, social patterns make this the exception rather than the rule. The shift from dying at home to impersonal institutions has created distance between the healthy and those who are ill and dying. As the aphorism "Out of sight, out of mind" suggests, with death no longer seen, it is more readily pushed out of individual and cultural minds.

Scientific optimism. Prior to biomedical scientific advancements, there was essentially little choice but to accept illness and dying. With the rise of modern medicine came a drastic change in our ability to intervene in disease and thwart death, such as through discoveries of antibiotics, vaccinations, and anesthesia. With such socially and psychologically impactful events as the eradication of polio and a cure for childhood leukemia, hospitals heroically emerged as centers of biomedical technologies and of hope for continued progress to thwart death. Of course, though the biomedical sciences have eradicated much illness and suffering, the death rate for humanity remains 100 percent. Unchecked optimism in future biomedical advances can easily become a hope in humanity's ability to overcome death itself through science. Scientific optimism, though grounded in the reality of the wondrous medical advancements of the past century, gives seemingly rational grounds to deny death.

Rituals around death. When death was "tame," the body of the dead family member remained in the home for days. This allowed families the opportunity to witness and directly handle the body of their loved one. After the funeral, the remains would be buried in or near centers of community life (typically churches), allowing for frequent visitation.

> Mourners publicly grieved in ceremonial black or by wearing black armbands, sometimes for extended time periods. Such rituals normalized death, permitted lament, and invited extended bereavement. In the twentieth century, many of these social customs disappeared. As previously noted, 70 percent now die in institutions, where the bereaved see their dead loved one's body only briefly, if at all. Even when a person dies at home, the corpse is typically removed from the home in minutes to hours, not days. Rather than family members and friends handling their loved one's body, strangers take charge of the dead person's body. In contrast to the traditional mourning practices that often extended for months after death, recent psychiatric standards identify grief extended beyond two weeks as possibly a clinical sign of depression.[11] As part of the taboo, grief is a medicalized problem. Finally, there is the rise of cremation in the United States from 3 percent in 1960 to 60 percent in 2023 (estimated to be 81 percent by 2045). While there are many positive reasons for cremation, Ariès describes this shift as part of a cultural psychology aiming to eliminate the memory of the dead. Rather than burials in local graveyards where the dead can be visited in their resting place, remains are scattered or are placed in containers often hidden from view, enabling the living to more easily forget.[12]

In the twentieth century, social changes made death something people could easily ignore, both personally and as a society. These alterations alone helped turn death into a taboo topic. But there is an even greater contributing force solidifying death as taboo. Individually and culturally, our hope has shifted from looking toward an eternal future to focusing only on what we can gain in this present and material world. This reflects the spirituality of immanence, which we defined in the introduction.

However, our drive for eternity is primordial. Death threatens this fundamental human yearning. This fear of death is mostly unconscious. *It* is a deep psychological energy that cannot be mastered. The ancient philosophers knew this.[13] Ernest Becker, in his pivotal book *The Denial of Death*, discussed how people need connections to immortality that foster hope beyond the present life to overcome fear of death.[14] He argued that with the loss of religion, modern secular societies depend on diversions and repressive practices to mask the terror of death.

Most religions, including Christianity, address the ubiquitous fear of death by upholding hope beyond this present world. In contrast, secular cultures ground all human reality solely in the present material world. Lacking any hope after death, secular societies need a mechanism to overcome the natural fear of death. But lacking any reality beyond what the philosopher Charles Taylor calls "this immanent frame,"[15] secular societies have only one answer to the fear of death: denial.

But the human fear of death is a difficult emotion to squelch. As a result, in a death-denying culture there are a proliferation of escapes. These include various forms of media, drugs and alcohol, sports, hobbies, and pornography, to name a few. Teens average nine hours a day on screens. Retired people ten hours. Substance use disorders have dramatically grown in frequency and now account for most deaths among young people.[16] Secular cultures are also obsessed with activities that uphold the illusion of unending flourishing in this life, including pursuing physical health and beauty, gathering material possessions, and the building of financial security. Running from the reality of death—despite its continual pursuit—keeps the fear of death in the periphery of our individual and cultural conscious minds, even as it motivates frenetic subconscious evasive practices.

Another way people in secular societies can attempt to avoid facing death is by seeking fulfillment or meaning that will survive beyond their lifetimes. For example, one's children can become a means of finding an identity that continues beyond death. The rise of "helicopter parenting" may be driven, at least in part, by parents deriving their sense of meaning and self-worth from the legacy of their children.[17] Parenting becomes charged with intense energy and anxiety when a parent's sense of meaning and purpose hinges on their children's performance. However, parental self-identification with children places tremendous pressure on them to be carriers of their parents' identities. A systematic review of thirty-eight studies examining helicopter parenting found consistent associations with depression and anxiety in children.[18] Children can be burdened not only by their own questions of identity but also by the weighty expectations of their parents' need for transcendence. Such stressors may be contributing to growing mental health issues and substance use disorders and overdoses in adolescence.[19]

People also commonly seek external vehicles for self-transcendence, often through one's work—for example, personal achievements and the pursuit of power—believing they will leave a lasting mark on the world. Too often, however, this belief collapses when one discovers that their contributions are easily replaced by others or that their ambitions for lasting achievement and influence are thwarted or swiftly overtaken.

For earlier Christian societies, death was understood as a tragic consequence of sin but not the end of human existence. Even in the face of death, there remained a victorious hope—a glorious life with God beyond the grave. Such enduring meaning and transcendence did not need to be sought within the limits of this "immanent frame," for they were secure and attained through death in Christ. As Paul declares in 1 Corinthians 15:54–55, "Death is swallowed up in victory. O death, where is your victory? O death, where is your sting?"

In stark contrast, today's secular culture is bound within the suffocating confines of the "immanent frame." Here, death is seen as a final and terrifying end to human existence, stripped of any future hope and magnifying fear into existential dread. At the same time, death has grown increasingly distant from everyday experience, hidden from sight and mistakenly presumed to be conquered by biomedical science. The result is a widespread denial of death, expressed through distractions like media, substance use, and relentless busyness as well as the pursuit of external forms of transcendence: one's children, career, or other achievements. Yet none of these diversions can overcome the fear of death; instead, its relentless pursuit drives a dangerous cycle of distorted behaviors aimed at silencing its terror.

Sickness Brings Confrontation with the Fear of Death

When sickness comes, a wrench is thrown into the death-denying behavior cycle. Though medical technologies often resolve sickness and keep the reality of death at bay, inevitably a sickness comes that cannot be fully resolved by medicine. At that point, a conflict ensues. The instinct for death denial clashes with the reality of mortality, and the reality of death percolates into the consciousness of the sick person and those around them. For some, fighting the disease and staunchly hoping for a conquest through biomedicine (or, for some, through alternative medicines) provides a narrative that detracts from the overwhelming reality of death. Although the use of treatments to alleviate suffering and cure disease is commensurate with the goodness and sanctity of human life, this approach can also become a new psychological means of denying *It*.

As sickness persists and worsens, the sick person can experience a sense of diminished value personally and socially. Our culture puts supreme value on health and wellness, diminishing the value of those who are no longer healthy. Carol, a middle-aged woman suffering from metastatic cancer, described her experience while being admitted to the hospital in this way: "I feel like this place is telling me that all I am is a body full of tumors that are killing me." Carol was sharing how she viscerally felt devalued as a person by the people caring for her. This devaluing can occur even when acute illness has been overcome, particularly when marks of prior illness are readily visible, such as a prosthetic limb. Visible reminders of the fragility of life and the inevitability of death are not welcome in this culture. The woman dying of cancer in the hospital is a reminder to all of the presence of *It*, a reminder that often leads to distance and avoidance for a death-denying culture. Similarly, the prosthetic limb speaks to the chaotic onslaught of *It*, an unstoppable force that will take not just limbs but all of our bodies.

Patients who are nearing the end of life can slip into a kind of trance shaped by death denial. Arthur was one of them. Even when Pastor David gently invited him to consider the nearness of meeting his Maker, a short time before his death, Arthur could not bring himself to hear it. He listened only to those who supported his determination to stay alive, and he shut out anything that suggested otherwise. His deafness to the truth became harmful both to himself and to those he loved. He was so focused on surviving that he could not see he was dying.

Between Awareness and Awakening

Lois was in a very different place from death denial. She was deeply aware of her emotions and attentive to her own inner life and to those around her. She had already faced death closely through the loss of both her parents. She helped care for her father as he was dying, and later, in her late forties, she became the primary caregiver for her mother during her final years. Watching her parents die forced Lois to face death directly rather than avoid it.

Saying goodbye to them and laying their remains to rest on the small beach near her childhood home on the Boston Harbor marked her deeply. After her mother's death, Lois turned to dance as a way of carrying her grief. Ballroom dancing brought together physical movement, creativity, costume making, and relationships. She danced three to four nights a week and became highly skilled, finding connection and meaning there.

At the same time, her spiritual life remained underdeveloped. Lois had grown up in church and absorbed the faith of her childhood, but as a young adult she stopped attending. She continued to believe in God and trusted that this life was not the end, yet her understanding of God and the afterlife remained vague. She was not clinging to this life as if it were all there was, but neither had she entrusted herself to the Divine Lover of her soul.

Psychologists of religion might describe this as a form of religious ambivalence or latent faith, where belief is present but not yet integrated into thought or daily life.[20] It is the posture of an undecided soul, spiritually awake but unsettled. Lois was avoiding God, neither wanting conflict with him nor ready to surrender. When we met her, as she faced cancer, she was emotionally open and willing to engage reality rather than turn away from it, but she needed help finding her way to eternal hope.

Illness can collapse faith into despair, but often it awakens seeds of faith planted in earlier seasons of life or offers fertile soil for new seeds of faith to germinate. In this way, Lois lived in an in-between place. Her serious illness would soon press her toward deeper spiritual decisions and force her to step off the fence she had long occupied.

The movement from a "tame" to a "wild" death has resulted in rampant subconscious death-denial patterns within secular cultures. Since Christians believe in the assurance of deliverance from the power of death, Christian communities within secular societies need not suffer the same death-denying beliefs or behaviors. However, the story of Arthur belies this assumption. In the next chapter, we see *It* as taboo not only for Arthur but also for many within the Christian church.

Three

Religious Denial

> Jesus said that if you have belief the size of a mustard seed you can move mountains. I find myself asking, "Why not me? Why can't I be like the masses that were healed?"
>
> Richard, cancer patient

Richard's Fight

Richard was forty-six years old when he came to his first appointment at the cancer center. His diagnosis would prove life-changing. Despite difficult treatments, the experience deepened his relationship with God, strengthened his marriage, and gave him resolve to be more present as a father for his two young daughters. But this was only round one for Richard.

Three years after he completed his curative treatments, Richard's cancer returned. Aggressive chemotherapies failed. The cancer progressed to the point of causing severe pain and difficulty swallowing. His oncologist, Dr. Patel, offered an experimental drug therapy, and Richard agreed to proceed with the research study. He was advised first to undergo palliative radiation therapy to reduce his symptoms. He saw the radiation oncologist soon thereafter. She explained that two weeks of palliative radiation should give him relief from these symptoms. But Richard didn't even know what "palliative" meant. The physician explained that palliative radiation treatment aims to relieve symptoms of the cancer but does not aim to cure the cancer itself. Upon hearing this explanation, Richard replied, "To be honest, I don't like that sort of attitude, Doctor. We're going to kick this thing, and I need you to be on my team."

The day after this conversation took place, Richard was interviewed as part of our study on the role of spirituality in cancer. During the interview, he told the story of his powerful religious conversion when he was thirty years old, after which he found his spiritual home in a Roman Catholic parish. The congregation formed a strong spiritual community that nurtured his faith as he struggled with cancer. He said that after his diagnosis, both he and his wife became closer in their marriage, and they made Christ the "absolute center" of their lives. He then described his firm belief in God's ability to miraculously heal him with the quote starting this chapter.

Several weeks later, and after starting the experimental drug, Richard was admitted to the hospital due to severe symptoms related to progressive cancer. He was visited by Dr. Patel, who explained that the experimental drug was not working and that he had no further therapies that could help. He recommended that Richard consider going home with hospice care. After a long pause, Richard plainly said, "Dr. Patel, I appreciate all you've done to help me, but I think I should get a new doctor. I need someone who's not going to give up on me."

Theology of Death

For Christians, death is the "last enemy" (1 Cor. 15:26). Its ugliness was graphically and publicly displayed in Christ's death on the cross. But though lamentable, death was not the final word for Jesus. Three days later, the tomb was empty; Christ Jesus had risen as Lord of all. Ironically, what appeared to be the ultimate defeat was actually the very pathway to victory—Jesus's accomplishment of our salvation.

Consider the irony: Adorning the walls of homes as well as churches and hanging from ears and necks is the cross—once an instrument of brutal torture and execution. We don't decorate our homes with elegant guillotines or wear delicate gold coffins as jewelry. And even these pale in comparison to the cruelty and public shame of crucifixion. Yet this very device of horror has become the ultimate emblem of hope. The cross of Jesus proclaims that death is no longer our greatest enemy. In his dying, *It is finished*; death was defeated and transformed into the doorway to eternal life with God.

Like Jesus, we who follow in his path have hope in life *through* death. And though death by its outer appearance is rife with pain, sadness, and hopelessness, it is ultimately the pathway that brings us "home with the Lord" (2 Cor. 5:8). Strangely, it is through death and its annihilation of all finite earthly hopes that there comes the greatest of enduring hopes: the hope of eternal life and intimacy with God himself. This hope will "swallow up death forever" (Isa. 25:8) and utterly remove death's sting (1 Cor. 15:55). The apostle Paul goes so far as to say that "to die is gain" (Phil. 1:21) and that he even prefers death: "My desire is to depart and be with Christ, for that is far better" (Phil. 1:23). Paul is not calling death good or minimizing its grief, but rather, he recognizes that death in Christ is the passageway by which every believer is ushered into the comforting, eternal presence of God. Accordingly, Christians need not follow the pattern of our culture that fiercely holds on to life by denying *It*. Rather, Christians can accept death while still embracing life because we know that Jesus's death, and our own in him, is the way to ultimate, unending life.

As Richard's story exemplifies, however, faith in Christ does not always lead to accepting death or to dying with hope. A Christ-centered view of dying will be explored in part 2, but first, we will consider how Christians may adopt death denial as their approach to dying and the consequences of doing so. Research shows that, within a death-denying culture, faith can develop its own forms of avoiding death. Shaped by a secular worldview that rejects any reality or hope beyond the material, faith can be distorted, mirroring that same denial and obscuring the Christian hope of eternal life through death. Themes underlying this tendency for faith to lead to death denial, and attendant data illustrating them, include (1) lack of end-of-life planning, (2) beliefs tending toward receipt of aggressive medical interventions, (3) church community spiritual support and greater aggressive end-of-life care, and (4) pursuing life prolongation in dying and the good death.

1. Lack of End-of-Life Planning

Several studies suggest that people of faith are more likely to avoid making plans related to medical treatments after becoming seriously ill. One study by True et al. found that, among incurable cancer patients with life expectancies of six months or less, those who looked to God in their illness were less likely to create a living will (a legal document that specifies one's treatment preferences at the end of life) as compared to those not relying on God.[1] Christians were also less likely to identify a health care proxy (a legally appointed person to make medical decisions in the event the person is unable to do so). One patient explained her decision not to make future medical plans by saying, "When I first got cancer, I told the Lord, 'I don't know anything about this, so I'm turning it over to you—you take care of it.' And that's what I'm letting him do." Her words illustrate how faith in God can sometimes lead to facing incurable illness in a way that sidesteps the personal work of consciously preparing for death.

Similarly, in our multiregional US study, our research group found that patients with incurable cancer who identified as religious were more likely than less religious patients to prefer every possible measure taken to extend life.[2] Even after adjusting for possible confounding factors through multivariable analysis, higher religiosity was associated with six-fold greater odds of preferring aggressive medical treatments at the end of life. These patterns left our team both surprised and concerned, prompting us to dig deeper to verify the findings and better understand the reasons.

2. *Beliefs Tending Toward Receipt of Aggressive Medical Interventions*

In addition to lack of planning and preferences about the future, our research group found that faith in God shapes actual end-of-life medical decisions. In a study of more than three hundred terminal cancer patients, those who relied heavily on faith to cope with illness were three times more likely to receive intensive life-prolonging treatments, such as cardiopulmonary resuscitation (CPR), in the last week of life.[3] They were also twice as likely to die in an intensive care unit (ICU). These patterns held even after accounting for factors like age, race, and social support. Coping with terminal illness through religious faith strongly predicted choosing more, not fewer, aggressive medical interventions near death.

Though the aforementioned studies are from US contexts, the few studies available in other cultural contexts suggest a similar pattern. A study of 317 patients and their caregivers recently admitted to ICUs in Sweden, the Netherlands, the United Kingdom, the Czech Republic, Israel, and Portugal found 45 percent of religious patients and 37 percent of religious caregivers preferred all measures to extend life regardless of the patient's condition.[4] In contrast, only 30 percent of nonreligious patients and 18 percent of nonreligious caregivers preferred all measures to extend life in any patient condition. In a study of 297 parents of infants in neonatal intensive care units in Hong Kong, those who regularly attended religious services were five times more likely than nonreligious parents to want every possible measure taken to save their child's life, regardless of the infant's condition.[5]

Human life is undeniably a beautiful gift from God, worthy of preservation whenever possible. Yet it must never become our ultimate hope, overshadowing the life to come. What was becoming clear in our research, and in the work of others studying patients and outcomes, was that the more deeply Christian a patient was, the more likely they were to pursue every possible option to stay alive, even when their illness was terminal. This does not mean that all Christian patients choose aggressive medical treatments at the end of life; many choose more comfort-focused care, such as hospice. Rather, it means that compared to non-Christian patients, Christians are more likely to want, and receive, all medical measures to extend life even when facing terminal illness. Importantly, pursuing aggressive medical interventions or hospice care in the setting of incurable disease are nuanced decisions unique to each patient. However, for Christians with hope for life beyond death, we and other researchers expected more, not less, adoption of comfort-focused care. We had assumed that Christians might feel *more* ready to meet God, *more* accepting of their mortality, and *more* willing than nonreligious patients to recognize when they were dying. But the evidence challenged these assumptions. It led us to ask why faith might guide people in this direction.

As Richard's story illustrates, Christians may use their faith as motivation to prolong life on earth while neglecting to prepare for death and eternity. While Richard's blending of faith with death denial is an overt example, such denial often appears among Christians in subtler ways. How often do churches intentionally teach about preparing for death or cultivating virtues in the midst of illness and dying? Do congregations even desire such teaching or find it compelling? Too often, churches avoid deep engagement with the spiritual formation that can take place in illness and dying, at least in part, because death is an unpopular topic. Messages promising blessings and positive outcomes *in this life* tend to resonate far more within our culture. This avoidance reveals, at least in part, an underlying adoption of the broader secular culture's focus on "this immanent frame," along with its accompanying tendency to deny death.

We now turn to exploring further the important role church leaders and faith communities often play in providing spiritual support to ill and dying congregants and their impact on those who are dying.

3. Church Community Spiritual Support and Greater Aggressive End-of-Life Care

Christians facing serious illness often receive needed spiritual and practical support from their faith communities. Many congregants make important medical decisions with counsel from pastors or other supporters from their congregations.[6] Not surprisingly, we also found that Christian communities influence how ill congregants make medical decisions at the end of life.

A US study of 1,005 randomly selected clergy, most of whom were Christian, found that many held religious convictions about the medical care of dying congregants that may encourage continuing to fight illness even when it is terminal. These convictions included believing that God can perform a miraculous cure, which was held by 86 percent, and pursuing treatment at the end of life because of the sanctity of life, which was held by 54 percent.[7] As expected, clergy who held these beliefs were less likely to discuss with dying congregants the option of stopping medical interventions or moving to hospice care.

Studies show that dying patients who are well supported by their faith communities are (1) three times *less likely* to go into hospice care, (2) two and a half times *more likely* to receive CPR or to be placed on a ventilator in the final week of life, and (3) six times *more likely* to die in the ICU as compared to patients not highly supported by a faith community.[8]

Remarkably, the most-religious patients who received the strongest spiritual support from their congregations were *eleven times more likely* to receive aggressive medical interventions in the last week of life and had a twenty-two-fold higher likelihood of dying in an ICU.[9] These findings persisted after adjustment for the patients' own religiosity and medical preferences recorded at the initial interview. These findings suggest spiritual support by faith communities compounds the likelihood of receiving aggressive medical interventions among religious terminally ill persons.

This evidence also suggests that embedded within church support can be a primary emphasis on staying alive rather than preparation for and acceptance of death. The encouragement or implied recommendation is to fight. From this perspective, death appears to be interpreted primarily as defeat, rather than entrance into the eternal presence of a healing God. These findings additionally suggest that many church leaders and faith communities may be inadvertently contributing to a larger social pattern of death denial.

One final possible link between faith communities and the pursuit of doing everything medically possible, including aggressive care, is an unintended consequence of belonging to a strong and loving community who, in that love, resists letting the dying person go. Of course, Jesus calls us to be a faith community characterized by love for one another (John 13:34). At the same time, when churches surround someone with deep love and care during serious illness, this support can unintentionally contribute to death denial through care that solely focuses on the continual fight against disease and the pursuit of care. Understandably, the community longs to hold on, to protect life, and to do everything possible in the face of suffering. However, by only emphasizing the pursuit of life prolongation and neglecting other virtues such as preparation, this loving care can become imbalanced. The sick person, grateful for such care and bound by love in return, may feel a quiet obligation to pursue every available treatment. This dynamic did seem to take place for Arthur and Richard, who both had strongly supportive faith communities that did not address preparation, at least not until very late in the illness. In this way, even faithful and well-intentioned care can shape medical decisions that resist acknowledging limits. Love remains a gift, but without careful discernment, it can subtly encourage a functional denial of death rather than a faithful preparation for it.

4. Pursuing Life Prolongation in Dying and the Good Death

Does pursuing life in terminal illness, such as through aggressive medical procedures, preclude a good death? In the aforementioned national clergy study, ministers were asked if a good death is consistent with ongoing aggressive medical treatments or dying in an ICU. Most pastors answered that a good death was not connected to whether a patient received aggressive medical therapies while dying or if they died in the ICU.[10]

They argued that the pursuit of medical interventions in terminal illness can sometimes prolong life and allow for greater time for spiritual growth and service to others in the Lord. "To live is Christ, and to die is gain" (Phil. 1:21). Life as part of Christ's body in the world is good! Furthermore, the pursuit of aggressive medical therapies in dying does not mean one cannot simultaneously pursue spiritual virtues in death, such as seeking forgiveness and reconciliation. In fact, at times life prolongation might be necessary to allow sufficient time for important spiritual processes to occur. As an example, a previously healthy seventy-year-old woman dying of a stroke received aggressive medical therapies in an intensive care unit for a few additional days despite her doctors indicating that she would not recover. Ongoing intensive medical care was provided until family members, including one child who had been long estranged, could come to the bedside, experience a form of reconciliation (albeit limited), and "say goodbye." Aggressive medical interventions at times can serve good spiritual purposes.

However, the pursuit of aggressive medical therapies can often work against the conditions of a good death. When these treatments are in fact an avoidance of and denial of death, dying persons and the communities surrounding them lose opportunities to seek and practice spiritual virtues in dying. This was evident in both Arthur's and Richard's stories. Arthur, who came from a Protestant, Evangelical tradition, and Richard, who was Roman Catholic, each had strong faith communities ready to support their spiritual preparation. Yet most of the energy of these communities remained focused on continuing medical treatments. In Arthur's case, his church devoted much of its time to praying for a healing miracle, as he requested. Pastor David tried to gently redirect Arthur's thinking, but it was too late.

When the inevitability of death comes despite death denial, the dying person and the community surrounding them can experience greater suffering because of the dying person's increasingly intensive medical care and the lack of preparation. For example, the ICU setting often leads to greater suffering for patients and families, particularly through the traumas associated with such care. In a study of nearly five thousand patients who had received care in an ICU setting and survived, over half experienced significant psychological morbidity—including anxiety, depression, and post-traumatic stress disorder—in the first year following their ICU admission.[11] A study of over three hundred family members of COVID-19 patients admitted to the ICU found that 63 percent were experiencing significant PTSD symptoms three months after their loved one's ICU care.[12] Dying persons receiving intensive medical treatments at the end of life not only experience the physical traumas of such care (e.g., pain and discomfort with intubation), they also often experience isolation from their loved ones and communities because they are in medical settings. Furthermore, ongoing medical care requires enormous physical, emotional, and spiritual energies for dying persons and their supporters, a toll that often detracts from or even precludes the pursuit of spiritual virtues in dying for ill persons, their families, and faith communities.

These data point to the negative impacts of aggressive medical therapies for dying persons and their families. Even though not every religious person chooses aggressive medical therapies, death denial can lead to poor dying in other ways, as illustrated in the previous chapter by the story of Arthur (who ultimately died at home). Lack of preparation and reconciliation, lost opportunities for spiritual growth, and unresolved spiritual struggles can negatively impact both the dying person and their loved ones. Arthur's wife, Joy, relayed her own and her family's trauma related to Arthur's death denial and avoidance of preparation for death. She poignantly stated that Arthur's death "was a bad death." She continued, "Right before he died, Arthur said, 'I'm leaving a mess.'" It has required several years to heal those painful emotions and traumatized family relationships.

Unintentional Death Denial?

Taken together, these findings reveal a significant disconnect between Christian theology and its lived expression. Christians have the spiritual foundation to know wholeness and certainty in dying—the hope of eternal life made possible in Jesus. Yet too many believers approach the end of life in ways that do not reflect that foundation. Why does this gap exist?

One possible underlying influence is the Christian emphasis on prosperity, growth, and blessing *in this life*. This does not merely include a narrower group of churches who formally subscribe to prosperity teaching or the "health and wealth" gospel.[13] Many across denominations are understandably drawn to the positive message of an "abundant life" (John 10:10). Pastors are inclined to emphasize messages of faith, hope, and love that encourage their flock. Sermons stress courage and the victory of God against suffering and despair. Contemporary worship music focuses on hope and life, rather than lament or suffering. The broken are stirred to believe that a loving and powerful God being constantly *for* you (Rom. 8:31) means the promise of total restoration *now*.

An emphasis on having faith for divine, rich abundance gives hope to the sick and downtrodden. Consider just a few book titles of one popular Christian author: *Your Best Life Now*, *The Abundance Mind-Set*, *Empty Out the Negative*, and *Your Greater Is Coming*. These themes have powerful spiritual appeal to those who are suffering as they cultivate hope despite the negative forces—both within and around us—working against life. These hopeful themes are based in wonderful biblical truths, such as the promise that God is preparing for us good things beyond our imaginations (1 Cor. 2:9).

Such messages of positivity have a dark side when they solely emphasize *certain* positive results in this *present* life (e.g., material success and physical health). Of course, the reality of our day-to-day lives speaks another story. Businesses fail, tragedies occur, and despite earnest prayers, many do not receive healing miracles. Scripture repeatedly emphasizes the hardship and fragility that characterize our lives in this world. Life is a "mist that appears for a little time and then vanishes" (James 4:14). We seek victory against death, but then we are "outwardly . . . wasting away" (2 Cor. 4:16 NIV). In fact, based on our Savior's own description, the life of *all* who follow him is best characterized as self-denial and the bearing of a cross: "If anyone would come after me, let him deny himself and take up his cross and follow me" (Matt. 16:24).

A robust theology must walk on the knife's edge between divine abundance and human finitude. A theology of divine abundance stresses flourishing, overcoming obstacles, and experiencing healing *in this life*. "I will not bring on you any of the diseases I brought on the Egyptians, for I am the Lord, who heals you" (Exod. 15:26 NIV). Yet hopes in this life must be balanced with a theology that recognizes our frailty and limits. Even when people earnestly pray for relief from chronic pain, mental health struggles, or disabilities, God sometimes responds, "My grace is sufficient for you, for my power is made perfect in weakness" (2 Cor. 12:9). And no matter how healthy we seem, we are all called to pray, "Teach us to number our days that we may get a heart of wisdom" (Ps. 90:12).

Living in the Balance

The empirical evidence and the experiences of Arthur and Richard suggest that the Christian theological framework shaping how many believers approach the end of life can, at times, drift out of balance. Richard's difficulty accepting the reality of his dying, along with data showing higher rates of aggressive medical intervention among some dying Christians, raises questions about how faith is informing these decisions. In some cases, believers and faith communities may place greater emphasis on abundance and healing in this life than on the biblical call to number our days in preparation for, and hopeful anticipation of, eternal life. While this imbalance may initially appear to be purely religious in nature, closer reflection suggests that it is also shaped by the broader secular culture, with its strong focus on this world and its widespread tendency to avoid or deny death.

In response to the death denial that has weakened Christian understanding, we turn in part 2 to seven pivotal spiritual concepts informing illness. We consider the seven last words of Christ from the cross as a guide for the seriously ill and those who care for them. For centuries, Christians have turned to these words for wisdom in suffering and dying. Here, we listen to them within the realities of modern medicine and a death-denying culture, asking how they can help patients and caregivers walk the path of Christ with courage and hope as they journey home to God.

We've taken license to change the traditional order of these words to better follow Lois's story. Traditionally, the order is based on comparing the Gospel accounts and on whether each word was spoken before or after the darkness that culminated in Jesus's cry "My God, my God, why have you forsaken me?" (Matt. 27:46; Mark 15:34). We begin with this word, a question, in chapter 4 because suffering raises immediate and difficult questions.

The chapters that follow trace a pastoral journey shaped by Christ's words. Together, they offer a spiritual path that guards both patients and caregivers against the pressures of a death-denying culture and emboldens them to follow Christ on the journey of sickness and dying.

Part 2

Illuminating the Path with Jesus's Words on the Cross

Four

The Silence of God

My God, my God, why have you forsaken me?

Mark 15:34

The one who does not see God's suffering does not see his love. God is suffering love. So suffering is down at the center of things, deep down where the meaning is. Suffering is the meaning of our world. For Love is the meaning. And Love suffers. The tears of God are the meaning of history.

Nicholas Wolterstorff

LOIS STARED OUT the large window next to her hospital bed. Snow mixed with rain fell soundlessly across the window of her sixth-floor room. The pain medication dripping through her intravenous line blurred her thoughts. The silence was broken by a knock at the door. Lois slowly turned her head and called out weakly, "Come—"

She stopped short when she saw the young resident doctor was already approaching her bed. The doctor was covered by a pale-yellow gown, a teal N95 mask obscuring her face and bright pink translucent glasses framing her eyes.

Her arms crossed over her chest as she began speaking. "Ms. Meinhardt, your MRI just came back and shows you have a tumor in the L4 area of your spine compressing your spinal nerves. You may need surgery, so we're asking the spine surgeons to come to see you. They should be here later this afternoon."

Lois looked at the young doctor for a long time. She slowly gathered the meaning of the words she had heard and then responded, "What's the 'four area' of my spine—is that bad? And I just had surgery to remove my kidney cancer a few months ago. Why do I need another surgery?"

The resident uncrossed her arms and motioned to her own low back as she spoke. "Ms. Meinhardt, there is a tumor in this area of your backbone, what's called the lumbar spine. The tumor is compressing your nerves, which is why you're having pain and trouble walking."

Lois interrupted the doctor, speaking somewhat frantically. "Are you telling me I have bone cancer now too?"

"No, no." The doctor shook her head, as if in reassurance. "This is the same cancer. It's now spread to your back. Like I said, we're asking the surgeons to come to speak with you about surgery. I'll be back later once they've talked to you. Is your pain better with the changes to your medications we made this morning?"

Lois nodded. "Yes, it's much better, though I'm very sleepy."

"Good," she abruptly replied. "I have to go now, but I'll plan to see you later this afternoon after the surgeons talk to you." She was already walking through the door as she finished her sentence. The door clicked shut behind her. Silence returned.

Lois looked out the window again. The doctor's name, which she had learned the day before, popped into her head finally. "Dr. Thayer," she said out loud to herself, testing her clouded cognition, something she did to pass the time. It was her second day in the hospital, and nearly all of her time was spent alone. With the COVID-19 pandemic, doctors and nurses kept visits brief, and she was not allowed visitors. She had received several calls from friends and new people from church who had befriended her since her diagnosis, but she had often been unable to answer, either because she was in too much pain or because she was asleep from her pain medication.

Lois looked at her flip phone and saw a missed call. She called voicemail to listen to the message. It was Martha, a kind, older woman at church who had been accompanying her to her oncology appointments. Martha had been there when Lois learned the cancer had come back just a week ago. Lois decided to call her back later. She would wait until after the surgeons had come.

Her mind began anxiously recalling Dr. Thayer's words. She looked down at her legs, bared below the hem of her hospital gown and still toned by years of ballroom dancing. But now, despite appearing strong, they were weak. She slowly lifted the left one, bending it at the knee, then her right. They felt like heavy weights were holding them down. Her legs awkwardly fell back to the bed.

Will I dance again? she wondered. *How will I pay my bills?*

Her ballroom dancing lessons had allowed her the little extra she needed to make ends meet. Though the COVID-19 checks were well making up for the financial loss of these last months, it wasn't clear how long those checks would last. But it wasn't primarily the loss of income that bothered her. She loved ballroom dancing. When she danced, she felt fully alive. Dancing had brought her through the years of grief after caring for her dying mother. She looked at her legs again, and her mind strayed to her last ballroom dance competition. She had worn a bright blue dress with a skirt that flowed in beautiful circular arcs as her legs masterfully moved in step with her partner and the big band music.

Was that my last dance? she wondered. Her chest felt heavy, and her back pain worsened as she pondered the question. She closed her eyes.

Her eyes tightened as more questions flooded her mind. *God, where are you? How could you lead me to this terrible place? How could you love me and do this to me?*

Lois felt panic welling up in her chest, then gripping her entire body. Her back began to throb again, and sharp, electric stabs of pain shot down her legs. She opened her eyes and fumbled for the call button. She found it in her crumpled bedsheet and pressed it.

Static sounded and a hollow voice came through the speaker. "What can I help you with, Ms. Meinhardt?"

"My pain is really bad," she said desperately. "Tell Sarah I need more pain medicine. Right away. I'm in terrible pain."

After a long pause, the woman's voice came through the speaker: "I'll let your nurse know."

The static cut off, and silence returned. Lois turned her head back toward the window to watch snow fall. After a long silence, she whispered, "God, where are you?"

Loss of Meaning

During stable seasons of life, we fill our days with meaningful pursuits and relationships.[1] We create systems of social connection, activities, and purposes that foster a sense of permanence and significance. When serious illness arrives, those stable frameworks of meaning are disrupted or even lost altogether.

When illness struck Lois, her life structures faltered. The loss of dance in particular triggered an internal crisis. Illness stole her primary way of coping through poverty, failed dreams, aging, and ongoing anxiety. Dancing had provided emotional and psychological regulation through artistic expression and exercise. With no more evening dance sessions during the week, she was cut off from friendships and her primary coping strategy. Lois's disease would eventually cause her to recognize that dance failed to provide the stable anchor she longed for, and ultimately, she would reevaluate what truly brings meaning.

In contrast to ephemeral systems of meaning, Christian spirituality offers a transcendent meaning-making system. Christian faith is built on the eternal, unchanging God who is an unshakable foundation. Many become more grounded in, or even discover, the bedrock of faith during serious illness.

Illness triggers a reorientation of priorities. During seasons of health and stability, many hold affections that are fleeting. But our life circumstances shift like shadows. Illness exposes inadequate affections that cannot withstand life's tumult. Career ambitions, romance, sports, money, and the arts prove transitory. Illness reveals these inadequate "little gods." One dying patient said, "Cancer is the best thing that has ever happened to me. Now I see what is important. I was too in love with small things."[2] Faith in God brings strength and clarity in contrast to lesser loves: "The Lord is a stronghold for the oppressed, a stronghold in times of trouble" (Ps. 9:9). Illness presses us to search for God, the only true, sturdy source of meaning.

The Silence of God

At the same time, faith can also lead to an opposite, negative crisis in illness. Illness and affliction may drive away all sense of God's closeness. When God feels absent, spiritual bewilderment and even rage can ensue. God's silence within affliction is a common complaint among the faithful:

> O God, do not keep silence;
> do not hold your peace or be still, O God! (Ps. 83:1)

> All our pleasant places have become ruins.
> Will you restrain yourself at these things, O Lord?

> Will you keep silent, and afflict us so terribly?
>   (Isa. 64:11–12)

> You who are of purer eyes than to see evil
>   and cannot look at wrong,
> why do you idly look at traitors
>   and remain silent when the wicked swallows up
>   the man more righteous than he? (Hab. 1:13)

In times of struggle, when we expect and most need God's voice and presence, the feeling of divine absence often terribly shakes the soul. Many see God's silence as more difficult to navigate than the actual illness or affliction. This is often, at least in part, because faith in God and his Scriptures yields an expectation of abundance and blessing:

> And the LORD will guide you continually
>   and satisfy your desire in scorched places
>   and make your bones strong;
> and you shall be like a watered garden,
>   like a spring of water,
>   whose waters do not fail. (Isa. 58:11)

When illness and divine silence are comingled, even the strongest faith can become bewildered and desolate. Such suffering is not foreign within Christian experience. Jesus, as he hung on a cross in physical and spiritual agony, cried, "My God, my God, why have you forsaken me?" (Mark 15:34). His cry is echoed down through the ages by Christian saints. In St. John of the Cross's classic *The Dark Night*, he poetically and theologically explores the suffering of the soul as it moves through the "dark night."[3] He describes this paradoxical experience as a "ray of darkness," because God's presence in suffering is a light so strong that it blinds the soul and reveals how little we understand. It is like stepping into the bright afternoon sun after sitting in a dark room for a long time. Initially the sunlight feels blinding not because it is dim but because our eyes are overwhelmed. In the same way, when a soul faces deep suffering, it can feel as if God is absent. Yet what is actually happening is that the soul is overwhelmed by God's presence; we are facing so much light that we think it is dark, so deep a presence that we mistake it for silence.

Suffering in the silence of God not uncommonly leads to rage, confusion, and self-accusation. In one study of seriously ill cancer patients, 30 percent wondered why God had allowed their cancer to happen.[4] Similarly, 29 percent were wondering if God had abandoned them. Among all cancer patients, 58 percent indicated some form of divine struggle, signaling that their connection with God was disrupted. When the ill face ongoing spiritual struggle, they experience greater depression, anxiety, and other mental health conditions. Several studies have reported correlations between spiritual struggles and greater physical pain, higher rates of suicidal ideation, and worse quality of life.[5] Studies have also demonstrated that patients with higher levels of spiritual struggles at baseline have a greater risk of mortality.[6]

In a qualitative study of family caregivers of seriously ill patients, caregivers expressed feeling exhausted, underappreciated, confused, and abandoned by God. "I am extremely angry with God," one caregiver expressed. "God kind of went over the edge on this one. This is clearly more than people should have to deal with."[7] Spiritual struggles with God in illness—for both the ill person and those caring for them—are common and are associated with poor psychological and physical well-being.

A Theology of the Suffering God

Scripture upholds faithfulness in affliction as being characterized by confident expectation of God's soon intervention: "He delivered us from such a deadly peril, and he will deliver us. On him we have set our hope that he will deliver us again" (2 Cor. 1:10). However, when Lois and others instead experience God's ongoing silence, they are shaken to the core. How do we accept God's silence?

Responding to this problem, theologian Jürgen Moltmann explores in his writings how God's silence is often misunderstood. He reasons that the presence of God is uniquely in the silence itself. God often does not swoop down like a superhero to pluck us out of our suffering. The nature of salvation requires that God enter the misery with us. God saves flesh by taking on flesh in the incarnation. Jesus undoes our suffering by entering the suffering. Moltmann says, "The suffering of abandonment is overcome by the suffering of love, which is not afraid of what is sick and ugly, but accepts it and takes it to itself in order to heal it."[8]

God's first necessary action of salvation for the afflicted was not to pull out the sufferer from his or her suffering but rather to bind his Spirit to the sufferer's spirit. By joining with the afflicted person, our suffering becomes shared with God. Rather than inflicting divine abandonment or rejection, the Spirit of God cojoins himself to the afflicted in solidarity. Though difficult to recognize, the Spirit of God experiences the divine silence with us.

This is a crucial mystery revealed when God in Christ suffered on the cross: "And at the ninth hour Jesus cried with a loud voice, 'Eloi, Eloi, lema sabachthani?' which means, 'My God, my God, why have you forsaken me?'" (Mark 15:34). At the cross, God is torn away from God into the silence of utter separation. Simone Weil described it this way: "This infinite distance between God and God—the supreme tearing, agony that no other has approached, marvel of love—is the crucifixion. Nothing could be further from God than the One who was made a curse."[9] Within the perfect unity of God, suffering, brought on by evil, rips God's nature asunder. In this mystery of affliction, God is forsaken by God. The enigma of the cross is that on the one hand, God distances himself from the one under the curse brought on by sin and subsequent affliction. This is an act of judgment and separation. On the other hand, God is himself the Afflicted One experiencing his own divine silence and abandonment. In the mystery of the Trinity, God suffers the silence of God. Thus, our perception of God's silence and abandonment in our experience is paradoxically connected to our unity with Christ in suffering. "Do you not know that all of us who have been baptized into Christ Jesus were baptized into his death?" (Rom. 6:3). Because we have been joined to Christ, the Spirit of God moans and cries out in unity with the afflicted, "Why have you forsaken me?"

Not only does Christ bind himself to us in our suffering, and in so doing suffer with us, but also the sufferer, in the affliction, uniquely enters and is bound to Christ's eternal suffering on the cross. In the suffering, the faithful afflicted is fulfilling Jesus's command to "take up his cross and follow me" (Matt. 16:24). Furthermore, in entering into Christ's eternal suffering, the sufferer—as a member of Christ's body—is uniquely bound to the atoning work of Christ's death on the cross:

> Now I rejoice in my sufferings for your sake, and in my flesh I am filling up what is lacking in Christ's afflictions for the sake of his body, that is, the church. (Col. 1:24)

The suffering person is mysteriously bound to Christ. Christ binds himself to and suffers with the afflicted. Simultaneously, the afflicted person, through their suffering, is bound to the eternal suffering of Christ—the selfsame suffering that conquers sin and death. These mysterious theological realities begin to unlock the unsearchable spiritual meaning and power within the lonely dark night of illness and divine silence.

Walking with Those in the Silence

In the same Boston hospital where Lois lay alone, Dawn also entered spiritual crisis. The two could not have been more different in their life situations, yet they both found themselves facing the same dark silence. Just prior to her hospital admission, Dawn's life was shattered when her husband tragically died without warning from a ruptured cerebral aneurysm. Because he died just three weeks after their joyful wedding celebration, Dawn regathered with many of her wedding guests for a funeral. His casket sat in the exact location where they'd exchanged their wedding vows.

Then two weeks after the funeral, Dawn was struck by sudden weakness and severe nausea. Tests revealed a serious bone marrow disorder that required immediate care. She began a long course of treatment that included frequent blood and platelet transfusions to keep her stable, followed months later by a bone marrow transplant once a suitable donor was found. She spent several months in the hospital, and it was more than eighteen months before she was strong enough to return to work.

Three years later, Dawn was still lost in the questions "Why?" and "How could God stay silent?"

"I do not understand what has happened to me. It is like God has shriveled me up and placed a target on my back," she told her pastor.

Her words echoed those of Job: "He set me up as his target; his archers surround me" (Job 16:12–13).

"Where do you think God is in all that has happened?" asked the pastor.

Dawn replied, "Every time I try to connect with God, all I feel is agony and then fury. As I try to pray, I eventually find myself screaming at him. The sweetness of the relationship has left me. It is like I've lost my innocence. I feel none of his kindness like I once did. I can barely bring myself to pray anymore. I end up hollering every time, which I don't like. His silence is cruel."

"Even if it is screaming, what do you say to him?"

"I'd rather not repeat it," Dawn admitted. "I don't normally talk that way."

Reassuring her, the pastor said, "Whatever you say, I'm sure God can take it."

"But why is he so silent?" Dawn stiffened, intensity rising in her voice.

"Are you sure God has been silent?" asked the pastor.

"I hear nothing! After all this time, I've tried to be faithful. Yet he has given me nothing."

Dawn stopped herself abruptly when, to her shock, she noticed tears were welling in the pastor's eyes.

He wiped his eyes with his napkin and said, "I'm so sorry, Dawn. It is so painful."

And soon, they were both crying. Dawn shared that she hadn't been able to shed tears for many months.

After a few minutes, the pastor continued. "Have you ever considered that perhaps the words of anger and fury that you are speaking against God are actually the Spirit of God speaking anger through you?"

Dawn was surprised and confused by the question. "I don't understand."

"You have said that God is far off. I'm not so sure. I believe that God hates the death of your husband. His heart is broken by the loss of your marriage. He despises your cancer. What if the anger that bubbles up in you is actually the Spirit of God expressing himself through you? Have you considered the possibility that your feelings of fury are actually some grace of the Spirit, who is permitting you to feel a tinge of all he feels about evil and death and cancer?"

With a puzzled expression, Dawn mused, "I've never considered that. How could that even be?"

"It just seems to me that the emotions you are feeling are similar to what we see in Jesus toward sickness [Matt. 14:14], bereavement [Luke 7:13], death [John 11:38], and especially bewilderment at his Father's silence [Mark 15:34]."

Continuing, the pastor said, "If what I am saying is true, it means that the Spirit of God has been much closer to you than what you have perceived. You've wanted a relationship of sweetness. We all desperately want this. But God is not just sweet. He is a Warrior who hates evil. God is a mystery that defies our small categories. You have lost a degree of innocence about God. Yet maybe God is permitting you to experience more of him, like when Moses saw his back side. To sense within yourself something about how God feels about injustice, evil, and death. This is no ordinary revelation."

"This has never occurred to me before," Dawn admitted.

"I know you've been told that your life has been a lot like the life of Job. It is a difficult gift to receive. At the very end, Job says to God, 'I had heard of you by the hearing of the ear, but now my eye sees you' [Job 42:5]. His severe suffering led to new revelation. And as it turns out, though God was silent for way too long in our estimation, Job was never alone."

Dawn's expression subtly lightened. "Thank you, Pastor. I've heard a new perspective today. I'm going to try praying into these things."

Faith Sees the Suffering One

Not only is it important for those suffering from illness to find God within their experience; family caregivers and clinicians must also see God within the sick. One of the great temptations in being around illness is to stop seeing the person. Exhaustion, burnout, and objectifying the sick are constant risks for those caring at the bedside. Family caregivers and clinicians can tend to distance themselves from the ill person because suffering is a reminder of their own vulnerability and finitude. At times, this distancing can go even further, leading them to see themselves as more important than the patient, since their skills and authority seem essential for the patient's well-being.

For example, the clinician might consider him- or herself to have superior or even godlike status in contrast to their patients because of their unique ability to save ill persons from life-threatening disease. However, Jesus's words in Matthew 25:37–40 aver the opposite—that the very presence of God is to be received in the sick person. We may go as far as to say that the healthy *need* to tend to and visit the sick as part of their own salvation. When we dismiss, avoid, escape, objectify, or grow tired of the sick, the caregiver's heart is revealed. The future judgment is tethered, in part, to how we see and treat the sick in our day-to-day lives (Matt. 25:41–46).

Lois often expressed frustration with the hospital staff because some were quick to leave her room, like the medical resident, while others were slow to respond to her requests, like her nurse. She was a very anxious person, and her anxiety sometimes left those caring for her feeling understandably exasperated. At the hospital, the medical team openly identified her as a "difficult patient." Demanding patients are the easiest for us to quickly dismiss, escape, or avoid. Yet Jesus made no distinction between demanding or grateful patients. "The righteous will answer [the king], saying, 'Lord, when did we see you . . . sick or in prison and visit you?' And the King will answer them, 'Truly, I say to you, as you did it to one of the least of these my brothers, you did it to me'" (Matt. 25:37–40).

Jesus identifies with the sick. Christ considers our being present with the sick as if we were visiting him. The suffering Messiah mysteriously connects himself to the weak and suffering.[10] Jesus reverses the stigma of illness. Rather than suffering meaning an abandonment by God, the Suffering Servant is bound to and hidden within the ill person. The sick are a sacrament of the Christ.[11]

Many Christians have responded to Jesus's teaching quite literally. Ancient monastic communities, for example, took meticulous preparations to welcome and honor the sick. Some monks studied and mastered the arts of medicine to be healers of both body and soul. If a sick person presented in need, the entire community would gather before the sick patient, bowing their faces in the dirt. They saw the holy presence of the Suffering One uniquely in the presence of the sick. Among the monks, a humble and hospitable concern for the sick "must rank above and before all else," including liturgies, community worship, or spiritual practices.[12] One cannot seek and see God without a heart of care and patience toward the suffering sick.

A Divine Invitation

Serious illness tests the soul, whether we are the ones suffering or the ones caring for the afflicted. The sick person must face the painful loss of worldly hopes and attachments. The dark night—the silence of God—can make suffering feel overwhelming. But Christian faith offers us a way through this experience. The word of Jesus from the cross, "My God, my God, why have you forsaken me?" reminds us that God himself cries out with us in that silence.

For the healthy caring for the sick, caregiving forces a confrontation with their own fragility and limits. This is difficult, especially in a culture marked by death denial, where the suffering of others is avoided to obscure the reality of our mortality. Yet what happened to Lois, Dawn, and so many others will, in one way or another, happen to each of us and to all whom we love.

At the heart of illness, affliction, and dying is a divine invitation to both sufferers and their companions to discover, in faith, the mysterious and suffering Christ. Faith within the silence and seeming absence of God is a crucial step into the very heart of God.

Five

Preparing and Planning

When Jesus saw his mother and the disciple whom he loved standing nearby, he said to his mother, "Woman, behold, your son!" Then he said to the disciple, "Behold, your mother!" And from that hour the disciple took her to his own home.

John 19:26–27

Teach us how short our lives really are
so that we may be wise.

Psalm 90:12 NCV

Advance care planning, even while it may unnerve us, grants us an avenue for worship through faithful discernment before catastrophe wrenches speech, thought, and prayer from us.

Kathryn Butler

LOIS'S EYES FLICKERED OPEN. A gowned, heavyset woman was next to her bed, adjusting the loudly beeping machine on her IV pole.

"What day is it?" Lois whispered in a raspy voice. The fog of heavy pain medication had lifted, and her mind was clearing.

"It's Monday," said the medical assistant with a thick accent that Lois couldn't place. The machine continued its beeping despite her efforts. "I'm gonna get your nurse." The door clicked shut as she left the room. Loud beeping continued.

Lois closed her eyes as she tried to put together how long she had been in the hospital. She'd arrived late on a Tuesday from the rehab facility. She was in the emergency room hallway for over a day before they brought her to her hospital room. Then she went to the operating room to fix her broken arm on Thursday morning. She realized she had been in the hospital for nearly a week.

A young man came through the door wearing a pale-yellow gown and teal mask, clearly in a rush. "Good morning, Ms. Meinhardt. Good news! I think we're going to be getting you out of here pretty soon."

"Hello, are you the doctor?"

"Dr. Coles—I'm the orthopedics resident who assisted your surgeon, Dr. Hui. Let me look at your incisions."

He was already reaching over with his bright purple gloves and undoing the snaps from her gown to bare her arm and shoulder. He looked at the incisions with apparent satisfaction.

"Incisions look great. We'll be getting you back to your rehab in no time. Probably sometime later today." He started moving toward the door.

Lois's voice trembled as she called out, "What do you mean I'll be leaving? I just had surgery. I need more time to recover. When I had my spine surgery, I was in the hospital for over two weeks. And I will *never* go back to that rehab. I had to call 911 because they wouldn't come when I called them over and over in pain from my broken arm."

Dr. Coles stopped in front of the door and turned toward her. "I'm sorry to hear about that, Ms. Meinhardt. This surgery is fairly simple compared to your spine surgery and usually patients get out within a few days. We're screening you for rehabs now, and you can let them know you don't want to go to the same place. The case manager will come by today." Dr. Coles quickly slipped through the door. At the same time, George the nurse maneuvered around him and entered.

"Good morning, Ms. Meinhardt. How are you doing? I see you're awake. How is your pain?"

"My arm hurts. It's a seven," Lois said reflexively before curtly adding, "I'm not going back to that rehab. They were awful."

"You won't necessarily be sent to the same place," George said reassuringly. "Janice, the case manager, will come by, and you can tell her you didn't like your prior rehab. Also, your rehab stay will probably be much shorter this time than after your last surgery. This is a much easier procedure." George adeptly opened the IV machine that had been beeping, made a quick adjustment, then closed it again. The beeping stopped. "I'll be back later with your pain medication, Ms. Meinhardt." The door clicked shut as he left the room.

Janice came a few hours later, awakening Lois from the sleep brought on by her pain medication.

"Hello, Ms. Meinhardt. I'm Janice, your case manager. How are you feeling today?" Janice, also covered in a mask and gown, dragged the chair from the corner of Lois's room to the small space next to her bed. She situated herself and began, "I wanted to review with you your rehab options. I'm thinking we can send you back to Hope House. They have a bed available today."

Lois interrupted her. "I will not go back there. They were terrible to me. I had to call 911 because they wouldn't answer my call button and turns out I had a broken arm." She motioned to her bared right arm with the healing incisions.

"Oh, I'm sorry, Ms. Meinhardt. I can look into other options. There may be one or two others that provide rehab and hospice care that we can consider, but I'll have to check what works with your insurance."

"What do you mean by hospice? Nobody has mentioned hospice before. I know what hospice is. My mother and father were on hospice when I took care of them." Lois was visibly angry as she spoke.

Janice looked taken aback. "Your doctors asked me to look into skilled nursing facilities that have both rehab and hospice. Has nobody talked to you about that?"

Lois snapped back, "Hardly anybody has talked to me since I got here, and now all of a sudden I have to leave when I'm not ready."

"It sounds like I should talk to your doctors and get back to you later, Ms. Meinhardt." Janice got up from the chair. "Hope you're feeling better. I'll be back soon once I understand more about your discharge plan."

The door clicked, and Lois was alone again. Her anger cascaded into incessant thoughts. *Hospice? Am I dying?*

She hardly slept that night. She repeatedly pressed her call button throughout the night to receive more pain medication. A soft knock awakened Lois the next morning. A masked and gowned woman peered through the partially opened door. "Ms. Meinhardt, is it okay if I come in?"

Lois answered sarcastically, "Do I have a choice?" Without answering her question, the physician came into the room and sat in the chair left by Janice the afternoon prior. She was silent for a moment before speaking.

"Ms. Meinhardt, I'm Dr. Spencer from the palliative care team. How are you doing this morning?"

"Not good. My arm is killing me, and they're making me leave the hospital."

Dr. Spencer, speaking slowly and taking notes, proceeded to ask Lois a number of questions. Lois answered with terse responses.

Finally, Lois interjected, "Dr. Spencer, I've been asked these questions many times before. Can't you just look in my chart?"

Dr. Spencer put her pen down and looked up at Lois. "Ms. Meinhardt, I've read your chart. I'm asking these questions to try to understand you and your situation a bit better. Why don't I give you an opportunity to ask me some questions. Do you have any questions for me?"

Lois looked past her. After a long pause, she asked, matter-of-factly, "Am I dying?"

Dr. Spencer adjusted herself in the chair. "That's an important question, Ms. Meinhardt. Before I answer, it would help me to hear from you what you understand about your illness. Can you share with me what you've been told so far?"

"I know my kidney cancer keeps coming back. Two months ago, it spread to my spine, and I had to have surgery. I was just starting to recover from that when cancer went to my arm and caused it to break. Doctors have told me it's in other bones and growing in my lungs too. When I saw my cancer doctor, Dr. Gillis, a few weeks ago, she said she would like for me to do a new experimental drug, but she wants me up on my feet again before we try another chemo pill. I was just starting to walk with a walker when this happened. I feel like we're playing Whac-a-Mole, chasing cancer spots as they come up."

Dr. Spencer paused before responding. "I'm sorry this has been so hard for you, Ms. Meinhardt." She remained silent for another few seconds before speaking again. "I did have a chance to speak with Dr. Gillis. We are worried that the cancer is moving fast and that your time could be short. She isn't sure if you will qualify for the clinical trial drug given how deconditioned you are. So, we need to make a decision. Either you can choose to stop cancer drugs and go on hospice care, or we could send you to rehab and see if you can get strong enough to be able to go on the clinical trial and receive the new chemotherapy drug. Do you have any thoughts about that?"

"I need time to think," Lois responded, "and I need to talk to my pastor and his wife."

Faith and Coping

Lois was overwhelmed and angry. Her health status was changing rapidly. Major health issues and related decisions—an initial cancer diagnosis and treatment, then a metastatic cancer diagnosis, back-to-back emergency surgeries, considering a clinical trial drug, and now a question about hospice care—were pummeling her wave after wave. It triggered more anger and new fears.

Serious illness is like traversing a field of land mines ridden with difficult emotions and complex decisions. During illness, we long to get better, maintain hope about the future, and receive optimal care. However, the unpredictability of the illness trajectory and the complexities and limitations of medical care often render these goals elusive. *Coping* refers to how one attempts to manage these challenging situations, their unknowns, and the waves of thoughts and emotions that attend them. To cope with stressors such as illness, multiple strategies can be employed. Depending on personality type and past patterns of behavior, certain strategies will be favored over others. Coping strategies are in part grounded in the truths of the Bible, but they can become sources of distortion when applied without their proper balance and prioritization in light of Scripture. For example, anger—a coping mechanism that Lois would often revert to—is in part based in biblical truths. Illness and death are evil, and hence anger is, in part, a rightful response. However, it is not the *only* truth at play in illness. If anger becomes a coping strategy that negates other truths—for example, loving others, trusting God's sovereignty, faith in God despite circumstances—then what is a rightful response to evil becomes distorted and even sinful (Eph. 4:26).

Many people in the church follow two common coping strategies in the context of illness—self-efficacy and passive religious deferral.[1] Both can be helpful but can also be subject to distortions.

Self-Efficacy

One common response to the confusion of serious illness is for the patient or their family members to take command of the situation. This coping mechanism is termed *self-efficacy*. With confidence in one's ability to learn and problem-solve, illness is managed through a variety of plans, logic, and strategies. The strategy of coping through self-efficacy emphasizes the role of the patient (and/or a family caregiver) in taking charge of the situation. This approach within serious illness has many positives. First, it can be empowering to the sick and their caregivers, providing a sense of control amid the unpredictability of serious illness. Second, it can ensure the best medical care as it provides the motivation and skills requisite to navigate the complexities of and barriers within health care. Self-efficacy and its related pursuit of good medical care is also in keeping with embracing medicine as God's gift to humanity. The practice of scientific medicine is grounded in the order of God's creation together with his commandment to subdue creation (Gen. 1:28). Furthermore, our pursuit of healing when illness strikes is encouraged by Scripture (James 5:14–16).

However, as is a danger with any gift from God, the pursuit of medical care can become distorted. Self-efficacy unchecked can result in an all-consuming drive toward healing. As described in chapters 2 and 3, Arthur and Richard exhibited this coping strategy and how a singular focus on medical care can lead to a neglect of other spiritual goals in the setting of serious illness. With Arthur, when his pastor attempted to address matters of his faith near death, the gentle invitation fell on deaf ears. By contrast, the early Christians, while receiving God's good gift of medicine, warned that the pursuit of healing should not turn "our whole life into one long provision for the flesh" so that the sick fall under a "craze for bodily health."[2] This approach to serious illness often leads into death denial as the pursuit of medical care to preserve life eclipses any processing of the coming reality of death. Like it did for Arthur and Richard, an intense focus on fighting disease and restoring physical health can distort perspective on the reality of one's true medical situation. This coping approach risks pursuing physical health to the detriment of one's spiritual health and relationship with God.

Passive Religious Deferral

The polar opposite of self-efficacy is called passive religious deferral.[3] Rather than emphasizing power and agency to problem-solve, this approach places medical realities and decisions "in God's hands." As in self-efficacy, there are aspects of this approach that are good and biblical. God indeed is sovereign over our lives, and we are to trust him with everything, including our health. Consider Matthew 10:28–31, where Jesus implores his followers to trust him, even under the threat of bodily death:

> And do not fear those who kill the body but cannot kill the soul. Rather fear him who can destroy both soul and body in hell. Are not two sparrows sold for a penny? And not one of them will fall to the ground apart from your Father. But even the hairs of your head are all numbered. Fear not, therefore; you are of more value than many sparrows.

In this approach, the ill individual passively waits for God to intervene. As a form of religious coping, it offers an immediate sense of relief from anxiety. A patient may say, "God has me in his hands.

I do not need to think about it." It also provides a powerful justification for the sick person to postpone difficult health decisions. This coping approach can frequently be employed at different time points, including the avoidance of proper estate planning, delaying medical attention despite indications of illness, or waiting too long to opt for hospice.

The concept of religious deferral was measured in a multiregional study of 275 seriously ill patients. The study reported that 67 percent of patients agreed with the statement "My belief in God relieves me of needing to think about future medical decisions (e.g., do-not-resuscitate order or health care proxy), especially near the end of life."[4] An active faith in God's sovereignty provides comfort by reducing anxiety among those facing serious illness. Furthermore, Scripture cautions believers about presumptuous attitudes toward future planning (James 4:13–17; Luke 12:16–21). As one patient memorably said to us, "If God wanted me yesterday, I wouldn't be here today."[5] Emphasizing trust in God's goodness and love can redirect attention away from the uncontrollable and distressing realities of illness, offering peace and reassurance.

However, an unbalanced emphasis on religious deferral can lead to unintended and harmful consequences. When medical decisions are seen and approached entirely from the perspective of God's sovereignty, people may feel justified in ignoring the practical steps needed to address their illness. One clarifying question that pastors and others can ask to help discern this is "Have you heard clearly from God to *not* take action around your symptom or diagnosis or, if you are honest, is fear possibly controlling your decision or lack of decision?"

For example, a woman who discovered a lump in her breast chose to rely on prayer alone rather than seek prompt medical evaluation. She prayed earnestly for months, but the lump did not go away. Because she waited to take action, her treatment was delayed, allowing the cancer to progress and reducing her chances for a good outcome from treatment.

Faith in God does provide refuge from the fear and anxiety that often surround illness and medical decisions: "God is our refuge and strength, a very present help in trouble" (Ps. 46:1). Yet faith can mask unaddressed fear, becoming a way to avoid the reality of illness and leading to confusion and harmful delays. One study found that terminal cancer patients who coped by placing primary emphasis on God's sovereignty had poorer understanding of the incurable nature of their disease.[6] This misunderstanding led some to believe they had years to live when in truth they had only weeks or months remaining.

These kinds of cases are not uncommon. They remind us that faith and wisdom must work together as we face serious illness and seek to respond in trust rather than fear.

Shepherding Souls

Growing up in the Midwest, Helen was a devout Christian from early childhood. She was headstrong, independent, deeply prayerful, and committed to telling others about Jesus. She never married. During her thirties and forties, she worked as an administrative assistant for a Christian school. In her later years, she spent most of her time serving at church, doing everything from serving meals to the homeless to helping with the children's ministry.

Helen was poor and lived alone in a small, one-bedroom apartment under Section 8 housing. She was extremely private. Even as her health declined and she had increasing issues with mobility, she did not initially allow church members to visit or help her. Eventually, she permitted occasional visits and help with groceries, but only after much persistence on the part of a few church members.

In her early eighties, Helen's physical health dramatically

declined. Though church members were concerned for her safety given her poor condition, she continued to eschew offers of assistance beyond occasional visits and grocery deliveries. Church members took to checking in on her regularly, given their growing concern, and many times Helen would not answer the door. At one of these check-ins, the church member assigned that week to visit didn't get an answer to her knocks. Given that nobody had heard from her in a few days, she summoned the apartment manager to open the door. They discovered Helen face down on her apartment floor, incoherent, in pain, and unable to get up. She had likely been on the floor for two days after having had a stroke.

After her hospitalization, Helen was told that a nursing home was necessary for rehabilitation. Any mention of moving into the nursing home was anathema. She would emphatically insist that the Lord had assured her that she would be returning home soon. "I am perfectly able to take care of myself," she declared. However, her fellow church congregants knew that it was not feasible, and certainly not safe, for her to go home alone.

The pastor, who also was named her health care proxy, said, "I don't think her going home is possible, but let's wait and see if she regains strength. There is no point in arguing with her now. She can barely get out of bed."

Helen had a steady stream of visitors. She loved to pray and would have every visitor read a psalm to her.

"A Psalm of Ascents?" she would ask every time in order to ensure that the reader would begin aloud with the superscription at the beginning of Psalm 121.

Repeat visitors began to realize that Helen chose this reading not merely because it was her favorite psalm to have recited but for the benefit of her readers. She loved to talk about Scripture, Jesus, salvation, and updates on the health of other ailing church members.

As the months ensued, Helen's body weakened, but her iron resolve to go home was unshakable. Accordingly, she insisted that her apartment lease for the upcoming year be signed and paid.

"Helen, perhaps someone can bring you a coat, a blanket, some extra clothes, and your mail? We want you to be comfortable for your stay here at the rehab hospital," said the pastor.

"Oh, absolutely not, Pastor! I'm going home, perhaps tomorrow," she insisted. "As soon as I can walk up and down the corridors with the walker, the doctor promised that I would be allowed to return home. There is no point in bringing anything here when I'm going home tomorrow or maybe a bit later this week."

Seven months later: same room and the same conversation. Helen's body was visibly wasting away to skin and bones. She developed bedsores on her heels. She became increasingly confused.

After reading Psalm 121, sensing the window of time was getting small, the pastor pressed again. "Helen, I know this has been hard for us to talk about, but would you permit me to ask you about the future?"

"Yes," she said with some hesitation in her voice.

The pastor continued. "I want just as much as you for you to go home. But it is also possible that this may not be God's will. It's possible that the Lord may call you to his better home very soon. Are you ready to meet the Lord?"

"Oh yes!" Helen exclaimed. "My heart is ready to see my Lord and Savior."

Sensing openness, the pastor pressed. "Praise God! I sense that you are ready too. In regard to being ready, if you were to get really sick, would you want them to send you back to the hospital to receive treatment, or do you think it would be better to keep you here to provide more gentle care and aim to take away pain?"

She spoke resolutely with firmness in her voice. "The Lord is on his throne. The Lord will keep my going out and my coming in." She was quoting Psalm 121. "I don't need to worry about that. I'm tired now, Pastor, and I think you should pray before you leave."

A few weeks later Helen would sharply decline. The nursing home doctor and staff, unsure how to manage her ongoing refusal to address her decisions, contacted the pastor multiple times to get his assistance. But Helen remained adamantly against discussing practical matters surrounding her dying. After Helen was no longer able to make her own decisions, the doctor recommended to the pastor that Helen be placed on hospice care. After consulting with others on the team caring for her, the pastor—as the designated health care proxy—heeded that recommendation. Helen died less than twenty-four hours later.

Helen left no plans or funds for her burial and no clarity on what to do with her property. These decisions fell on a few committed church members. As they cleaned her apartment after her death, church deacons found several piles of hidden cash. It was stashed, a few hundred dollars here or there, and in dozens of letters hidden in the back of her bedroom closet. The letters sat in a trash bag, which could have easily been discarded but for patient and tender sorting of items. To everyone's surprise, she had enough funds to cover her remaining costs upon her death. All outstanding bills were paid, and her funeral expenses were covered. There were even some remaining funds, which were donated to support Helen's most beloved ministry efforts.

Helen's passive religious deferral was not something she could overcome in this life. Yet even then, grace revealed itself. Helen did arrive "home," just as she contended. Though she refused to plan ahead, God intervened. Psalm 121 was fulfilled: "The Lord will keep you from all evil; he will keep your life. The Lord will keep your going out and your coming in from this time forth and forevermore" (vv. 7–8).

Prudence

God's sovereignty is a powerful truth in which we find refuge, yet it does not remove human responsibility. Religious deferral can easily become an unhealthy way to avoid facing difficult realities and emotions, especially in a culture that often denies death. Faith in God's sovereignty, as seen with Helen, lessens anxiety and cultivates humble trust. However, trust in God does not eclipse the exercise of human responsibility through prudence. These two, faith and foresight, are meant to work together.

Through divine providence, God oversees, protects, and preserves life. Trusting in his providence means we do not have to be anxious about tomorrow (Matt. 6:34; Phil. 4:6–7) nor presumptuous about the future (James 4:13–17). We are called to accept the will of God, even when it is not what we would choose (Matt. 26:39).

Prudence remains a necessary virtue. As Proverbs 14:15 reminds us: "The simple believes everything, but the prudent gives thought to his steps." Thomas Aquinas, quoting St. Augustine, described prudence as "knowledge of what to seek and what to avoid," the foresight of one who "sees from afar."[7] The prudent foresee death, not with dread but with preparation, so that when they die, their loved ones are, to the degree that is feasible, not encumbered by planning matters the dying person could have undertaken. Bereaved loved ones are not only freed to grieve and tenderly remember, but they can also be blessed by the love and example manifest in the preparation.

Planning for future medical needs or estate matters should not be a source of anxiety. Rather, it is an act of wisdom and love. The prophet's call to Hezekiah, "Set your house in order" (2 Kings 20:1), remains a wise directive. Preparing for serious illness and death acknowledges life's brevity (Ps. 90:12) and offers a gift of care to those who remain.

Jesus himself models this kind of practical, tender love. From the cross, he entrusted his mother to the beloved disciple: "'Woman, behold, your son!' Then he said to the disciple, 'Behold, your mother!'" (John 19:26–27). Though Jesus trusted the Father completely, he still took tangible steps to ensure Mary's future care. Jesus would not die before clarifying certain wishes and passing on earthly responsibilities. Likewise, prudence foresees one's death; love for others prepares for it.

Setting Your House in Order

Medical Planning

Prudence anticipates medical decisions that may arise when one is too ill to speak for oneself. Preparing well requires asking thoughtful questions of physicians and other clinicians. Below are listed a few categories and questions health care initiatives recommend considering:

- Illness understanding and prognosis: "What is my current condition, and what can I expect in the coming weeks or months?"
- Choices: "What are my treatment options, and what are the likely benefits and risks of each?"
- Quality of life: "How will these treatments affect my daily life and ability to do what matters most to me?"
- Palliative and hospice care: "If I stop curative treatment, what kind of comfort and support will be available?"
- Medical burdens: "What are the financial, emotional, and physical burdens of the different treatments?"
- Professional advice: "Given what you know about my situation, what would you recommend if you were in my place?"

Choosing a health care proxy—someone legally empowered to make decisions if you cannot—is critical. A proxy must not act on their own preferences but rather honor the patient's wishes. While a living will provides helpful guidelines, complex medical situations often require personal judgment. Thus, conversations with a proxy are vital and considered more effective since living wills cannot anticipate every medical scenario.

Some questions to explore with a proxy include:

- Are you willing to undergo aggressive treatments if it might extend your life but with significant physical or cognitive limitations?
- Would you want life-sustaining medical treatments if there were little hope of recovery?
- In what situations would you want to stop aggressive medical treatments and allow natural dying to occur?

Earthly Planning

In practical terms, preparing for death includes:

- Providing clarity to the decision-makers and procedures after death through legal documents and designations (e.g., a will, trust, health care proxy, power of attorney).
- Providing clear instructions about funeral and burial wishes.

Thoughtful estate planning not only prepares for the future but can also ease the fear of death. A carefully crafted will or trust anticipates a range of outcomes and distributes resources with intention and love. In contrast, the absence of a plan can lead to family conflict, unresolved grief, and devastating legal struggles. Openly communicating your wishes, just as Jesus did, can help prevent division and confusion. If Jesus had not passed on the responsibility of care for Mary, it could have caused disagreement and strain among his followers and family. Instead, by clearly entrusting her to John, he protected them from this and gave us an example to follow.

Estate planning provides a powerful opportunity to leave a meaningful legacy by blessing children and grandchildren, supporting ministries or causes close to your heart, and lessening emotional and financial burdens on loved ones. Regardless of the size of one's estate, these final decisions can become intentional acts of love, offering thoughtful blessings to each person involved. Planning for bodily remains and offering guidance for a funeral or memorial service are also profound expressions of care, compassion, and mercy.[8]

Spiritual Planning

Even more essential are the spiritual dimensions of preparation, which inform and give deeper clarity to the practical steps of preparation just mentioned. Preparing for death can become a sacred opportunity to draw closer to God and to those we love by:

- Engaging in prayerful discernment about how God may be calling you to steward your resources after death, with careful attention to the needs of those entrusted to your care, such as family members or organizations.
- Seeking meaningful closure in relationships through intentional acts such as writing a legacy document that shares life stories and blessings, or having heartfelt conversations that express gratitude, uphold forgiveness, and affirm love.

Addressing these matters early, while still in good health, provides the time and mental clarity needed and reduces stress in the future. Postponing these conversations can lead to missed opportunities to bless others through practical preparation, to experience spiritual growth, and to strengthen meaningful relationships. It may also place a heavier emotional and practical burden on those you leave behind. To further help with this process, use the End-of-Life Planning Checklist in appendix A.

Advocates for the Journey Home

Lois had a difficult decision to make as she lay recovering from her arm surgery in the hospital. She was in pain and deeply anxious. COVID restrictions made everything harder. Most hospitals and rehabilitation centers would not allow—or greatly limited—visitors, and Lois feared being left alone again. Michael and others were calling on the phone, and while this helped, Lois needed someone present. By God's grace, I (Tracy), as a physician working in the same hospital, was able to visit her. This became a special grace, because I could see and understand Lois in ways the busy medical team had missed.

Lois had already endured a terrible experience in a skilled nursing facility. She had a broken arm from cancer that had spread to the bone, yet her pain was dismissed. She was left alone for so long that she finally called 911 from her bed. The staff had assumed she was confused or just difficult, but she was being neglected and was advocating for herself in the only way she could. That experience left her terrified of ever returning to a place where she would be unseen and unheard. When the palliative care doctor talked with her about further cancer therapy versus comfort-focused hospice care, Lois knew she did not want more cancer treatment. She wanted less pain and she wanted to be home.

Normally, a patient like Lois would be sent to a skilled nursing facility where hospice could also be initiated, and that is what the medical team recommended. But I could see that this would not work for Lois. First, the tight restrictions on visitors would render Lois largely alone—something she greatly feared. Furthermore, it was clear to me that Lois was someone who was highly sensitive emotionally and even physically, including having poor tolerance to the side effects of pain medications. But there was one option that would not leave Lois alone and would optimize symptom management: inpatient hospice.[9]

Inpatient hospice could provide the IV pain medications and careful monitoring Lois needed, and, most importantly, it allowed visitors during COVID, since patients were already understood to be dying. It offered what she longed for: comfort and the presence of people who cared for her. When I explained this option, the relief on Lois's face was evident.

The difficult part was convincing case management. Inpatient hospice beds are highly limited, and Medicare has strict rules for qualifying. Lois's chart, without her story, made her look like a routine patient who should go to a skilled nursing facility. As Lois's advocate, I met with her team and shared the fuller picture. I explained Lois's severe pain needs, her emotional fragility, her decision to stop treatment, and the great harm another stay in skilled nursing would cause. After several conversations, the case manager thought Lois could qualify and the medical team agreed that inpatient hospice was medically indicated.

Michael and I walked with Lois through the transition. At the hospice center, visitors were allowed, and her pain finally came under control. For a time, we believed her last weeks would be spent there.

Looking back, we came to see how much depended on advocacy, knowing the system, understanding Lois, and speaking for her when she could not. Many people do not have a physician directly advocating for them. In our national congregational survey, we found that churches average about two physicians and six nurses within their congregations.[10] Over the years, we have also walked alongside and discipled many hundreds of nurses and physicians, and while they are often very busy, we have found that when invited, many are willing to share their medical wisdom for the sake of their church community. Yet in practice, relatively few churches draw on these gifts to help guide others in advanced care planning or to offer support with medical decisions during serious illness.

Jesus's words from the cross, "Behold, your mother," remind us that he calls us to care for one another in this same spirit of watchfulness and responsibility. In moments of deep vulnerability, this kind of advocacy can be an instrument of Christ's love.

Avoidance or Surrender?

When Lois was confronted with her diagnosis, she chose a path of preparation and surrender. She allowed people to help her.

Helen, by contrast, could not bring herself to face these matters. She avoided every conversation about dying. Pressed by the hospital, she reluctantly named her pastor as her health care proxy, but she would not articulate any wishes to the pastor, despite his efforts to talk with her. As Helen's condition worsened, it was left to her proxy and physicians to intervene. Without a clear directive otherwise, medical staff are required to proceed with intubation and aggressive treatments, often leading to death in an intensive care unit. Fortunately, the nursing home staff working alongside Helen's pastor as her proxy advocated she receive hospice care, prioritizing her comfort over futile prolongation of suffering.

Two women walked two diverging paths. One chose to manage what could be managed and surrendered what could not. The other chose avoidance, and others were called upon to make difficult choices on her behalf. The Lord was clearly present for and blessed both of these dear ladies in their dying, even despite their weaknesses.

Serious illness brings not only medical challenges but also deep spiritual responsibilities. Coping strategies such as self-efficacy and religious deferral can serve us well, yet both require wisdom and balance. Scripture teaches that planning and preparation are not a lack of faith but important spiritual tasks modeled by Jesus himself when, from the cross, he ensured his mother's care. When faith and prudence work together, preparation becomes an act of love that honors God and protects those we leave behind. In the next chapter, we will discover that one of the most common reasons Christians fail to prepare for the future is by holding out hope for a miracle.

Six

Addressing Miracles and Fears

> And he said, "Jesus, remember me when you come into your kingdom." And [Jesus] said to him, "Truly, I say to you, today you will be with me in paradise."
>
> Luke 23:42–43

> God can do everything. He can raise someone from the dead if he wants. Yes, God can do a miracle. Don't be angry if he doesn't do a miracle because God's will is inscrutable. We don't know his ways.
>
> Eastern Orthodox priest, Boston

Uncle Mike's Peace

The first time I (Michael) witnessed what I consider a healing miracle happened around my Uncle Mike's death. My mother named me after him. He was my godfather and someone I admired. He taught me many things over the years, but it was during his final illness that I learned the most important lesson of all: what it means to be a pastor who stays close to someone in grave illness. This was the last lesson Uncle Mike gave me, and it was the most profound. Through that experience, God expanded my understanding of healing miracles beyond my narrower theological limits. His dying shaped how I came to Lois's story, because without it, I do not think I would have been open to welcoming her into our life. Through my uncle, I was given a larger vision of what God may be doing in the midst of serious illness and death.

Uncle Mike had always been strong. He co-owned a construction company for thirty years, and before that he worked as a welder. As a young man, he once fell off a ladder and broke his back and returned to work within two weeks. He was the kind of person who worked through pain and just kept going.

But this time was different. Now in his late sixties, he could not breathe. It was not age or a passing illness. He was diagnosed with mesothelioma, a cruel cancer that coats the lining of the lungs, which was caused by asbestos exposure during his years of welding and construction.

The doctors recommended surgery, a major and invasive procedure, even though the average survival was only twelve to fourteen months.

I visited Uncle Mike in the hospital about a week after that surgery. He was sitting in a chair when I arrived, smiling as the surgeon was just finishing his daily rounds.

"What do you think, Doc? How am I doing?"

"You're doing remarkably well for just seven days out. I'm very encouraged by your progress."

Uncle Mike turned to me and beamed. For a moment, it seemed like the Lord had breathed on him, and he was feeling like a new man.

"It's a miracle," he told me. "I thought I was as good as dead, but now . . ." He didn't finish the thought. He had stared death in the face and won.

When Uncle Mike was hospitalized at a major Harvard teaching hospital, he was cared for by surgeons known for bold and aggressive treatments of mesothelioma. These surgeons were spoken of with awe, almost as living gods, because they dared to operate with new procedures. Some patients lived far longer than expected, and a few of these surgeons became medical legends. For Mike, receiving their care brought real and genuine hope. He had a renewed sense that life might still be reclaimed where death had once seemed certain.

But both the surgeon's triumphant march and the cancer's reprieve would prove to be short-lived. Two months later, the call came.

"Uncle Mike is scared," my mom said, her voice cracking. "He's in the surgical ICU. I just spoke with him, and I can tell he's afraid. They're considering sedation. Would you please go and visit your uncle?"

Should I go now? I wondered. My house was just a seven-minute walk to the hospital. I was staring at a looming work deadline, blinking at the screen. My best writing always came in the morning. I had been focused and making progress just before my mother's call. I told myself I'd go at the end of the day. What's a few extra hours if I showed up later?

But unease settled over me. Ten o'clock passed. Then 10:15. I couldn't shake it. I knew this was a holy nudge. It came as an inner urge that I needed to forget writing and go immediately to the hospital.

I sighed, grabbed my Bible, and started walking. I didn't know what I was going to say. I had never been in a situation like this before. What do you say to a man standing at the edge of eternity but who has never before shown readiness to acknowledge it? The Holy Spirit often leads us into places that stretch us, but he also meets us there with special grace.

Uncle Mike didn't know it, but he had been surrounded by prayer for years. My mother, his older sister, had prayed for him for forty years. And then one of my sisters had her entire church praying for Uncle Mike's soul. We don't know exactly how, but there is a real and mysterious relationship between our prayers and the Spirit's actions.

When I entered the ICU, he was still conscious, though struggling to breathe. Machines beeped steadily in the background. My two cousins, his son and daughter, hovered nearby. Doctors moved in and out, discussing sedation. I watched him—his chest rising and falling with effort. Every breath was a battle as his lungs were failing.

The medical team heard I was a pastor and quietly stepped back, giving me space and a few moments alone with him. And then, something unexpected broke loose inside me. I began to sob. A deep, full-body cry. It caught me by surprise. I cared for my uncle, but this was something different. Not from fear or grief, but something beyond me. Later, I came to realize that it was the Holy Spirit weeping through me.

"I'm not dying yet," Uncle Mike whispered, almost defiantly, in response to my tears.

"I'm so sorry you're back in here," I said gently. "How are you feeling about all this?"

After a pause, he admitted, "I'm afraid. I could use a miracle right now."

I read Scripture aloud. He listened, though his breaths were short and labored.

Then, between gasps, he looked at me. "Maybe you have a few words that I can say?"

He wanted words to help him pray. They came immediately, from somewhere deeper than my conscious mind. I had read the words the night before, and as soon as he asked me, these words came rushing into my mind. It seemed again to be the Holy Spirit.

"Lord Jesus, have mercy upon me, a sinner."

He repeated, "Lord Jesus, have mercy upon me . . ."

Then silence. I waited, keeping my eyes averted. I sensed he was having difficulty admitting to himself, and to God, what those final words required. Something seemed blocked, as if a dam were holding back more than speech. So softly, I prompted him with no more than a whisper: "A sinner."

After a long pause, he whispered, "A sinner." His face twisted with sorrow and then relief.

When he finally said "a sinner," it felt like a dam had broken in his soul. Something important was released. At the moment, I didn't feel it was the right time to ask or press. Maybe I'd have another chance to visit tomorrow and talk more about what had happened.

When I said goodbye, he smiled weakly and there was something like wonder or surprise in his expression. Uncle Mike's last words to me were something I'll never forget:

"I feel peace."

At 1:00 p.m. that same afternoon, less than two hours after I left him, Uncle Mike was sedated. He never woke again in this life.

What if I had waited like I'd initially decided? What if I had finished my writing first and visited in the afternoon? What if those prayers over the years had never been lifted? But God goes before us. The Spirit woos the soul. And even in our hesitations and stumbles, he moves.

All we're asked to do is keep in step with the Spirit and watch the power of God unfold.

Uncle Mike asked for a miracle that day. Though it could barely be recognized with natural perception, I witnessed one of the greatest miracles of my life. I witnessed this man experience a healing miracle even as his body died. This early pastoral experience taught me—Uncle Mike taught me—that the Spirit does miracles in more than one way, and it is never too late to receive or be part of one.

The Divine Healer

God reveals himself as the source of all healing. "I am the LORD, your healer" (Exod. 15:26). He is a God of both mercy and power, who heals body and soul by restoring and making whole (Ps. 147:3). In the Old Testament seven healing miracles (Num. 12:1–15; 21:6–9; 1 Kings 13:4–6; 17:17–24; 2 Kings 4:1–37; 5:8–14; 20:1–11) occurred between the times of Moses and Elisha, which was approximately five hundred years. But when Jesus arrives as Messiah, there is an extraordinary increase in healings, as recorded in the four Gospels. Within just a three-year period, there are twenty-seven written accounts of healings in the Gospels, and at least thirty-six different persons healed by Jesus in those accounts. In addition to these specific examples, many others are said to have been healed by Jesus (Matt. 4:23; John 21:25). From a larger point of biblical history, Yahweh as Healer comes to earth in the person of Jesus, releasing an abundance of divine healing energies rarely witnessed in the Old Testament.

Why is there a mushroom of healing miracles connected to Jesus's arrival?

First, with the arrival of Jesus as the Son of God, there is a direct confrontation between good and evil as it relates to illness. Sickness is one of the hallmarks of Satan's grip over the world. His intention is to steal, kill, and destroy (John 10:10). With the arrival of Jesus, who is none other than Yahweh, the Healer (Exod. 15:26), the goodness and abundance of the life of God enters into the sickness of the world. When God's life encounters our world's death, the divinely animated powers of life come into full display. Just as darkness cannot withstand the light, illness cannot thrive in the presence of the Divine Life.

Second, with the arrival of Jesus and the Holy Spirit, the compassion and *agape* love of God are on full display. Jesus is angered toward illness, showing compassion to the sick. He has compassion for the dying (Matt. 14:13–14; John 11:32–37). The healing powers of Jesus are an expression of his deep love. The love of God in Christ cannot help but heal.

Third, the outpouring of healing by Jesus, and then later by his apostles, forms a proclamation and sign of the reign of God. Just as the ancient Jewish tradition of Jubilee freed slaves and forgave debts every fifty years (Lev. 25), Jesus declares a new and greater spiritual Jubilee, which includes liberty for the blind and sick (Luke 4:16–22). The overflow of healings in the Gospels is a sign that God's new kingdom and the favor of the King have now dawned. Of course, because these healings are signs, they are not the fullness of restoration. As VanderWeele reminds us, "Salvation does not, in this life, free the body from illness and death."[1] However, Jesus's displays of healing serve as previews and assurances that the full restoration of God's kingdom will be completed at the end of time.[2] We are now in the beginning of a new season of the Lord's favor.

Miracles in the Church

Jesus authorized a larger group of his disciples ("the seventy-two") to preach the gospel and to heal diseases (Luke 10:9). Some biblical scholars interpret a symbolic meaning of seventy-two to refer to the reversal of Babel (Gen. 11).[3] In Genesis, seventy-two nations were surrendered to dark, evil powers, whereas Israel belonged to Yahweh (Deut. 32:8). Through Jesus, all nations are being reclaimed by him in the sending out of the seventy-two disciples. The nations are shrouded in dark illness. Jesus's healing powers are granted to the church to proclaim the gospel to all nations. The signs of healing are a demonstration of the arrival of God's kingdom and the downfall of Satan (Luke 10:18). Healing serves as a tangible sign of Christ the King's eternal compassion and life. Thus, a central task given to the church is to bear witness through healing signs to the sick.

Unsurprisingly, throughout church history, miraculous healing has been both celebrated and contested. In the fifth century AD, St. Augustine famously abandoned his previous belief that miracles had ceased with the death of the apostles after witnessing a healing of epilepsy. During the final years of his life, he went on to investigate and confirm nearly seventy miracles in a two-year span in his diocese in Northern Africa. In *The City of God* he noted in great detail, and to the shock of the physicians, healings of patients with breast cancer, blindness, and an anal fissure. "The truth is that even today miracles are being wrought in the name of Christ," he concluded.[4]

Yet in the modern era, claims of healing have also produced serious distortions. Kate Bowler's study of the prosperity gospel shows how faith can be presented as a guarantee, bringing health and wealth to those who set aside biological and medical explanations in favor of supernatural causality.[5] Such teaching can cause real harm, especially when the sick are urged to refuse medical care or are blamed for a lack of faith when healing does not come. These distortions misrepresent God and burden the vulnerable with guilt and despair.

Setting aside prosperity teaching, there remains broad agreement across Christian traditions that God may still heal miraculously. Divine healing emphasizes God's freedom to heal as he wills, often in response to prayer and always as a sign of his goodness. Such healings are uncommon, not routine, and are meant to stir awe and point toward ultimate salvation.

Frequency and Temporary Nature of Miracles

Definitions of miracles vary. Sulmasy describes a miracle as a rare event that cannot be explained by ordinary means, evokes wonder, carries spiritual meaning, and is recognized by the believing community.[6] In medical contexts, investigations such as those at Lourdes often apply the strictest criteria: a verified diagnosis, an incurable condition, an instantaneous and complete recovery, and no medical treatment sufficient to explain the cure.[7]

Many Christians use the word *miracle* more broadly, recognizing God's hand at work in extraordinary recoveries, even when medical explanations remain possible. In a national clergy study, nearly one in four pastors reported witnessing a miraculous healing through prayer alone in the prior year. Most involved serious illness, especially cancer.[8]

No matter the definition, all bodily healing miracles in Scripture are temporary. Hezekiah was healed and given fifteen more years of life, but he still died (2 Kings 20:1–7). Lazarus was raised from the dead (John 11), yet his resurrection was, as Gaffin notes, "temporary and insubstantial."[9] Craig Keener similarly reminds us that "everyone dies," and that every remission, no matter how hopeful, is ultimately short-lived.[10]

This reality does not diminish our faith in the living God, who at times acts with extraordinary love and power. God may heal powerfully in this life, but death remains until Christ finally defeats it (1 Cor. 15:26). Pastorally, this means we must help people face their dying faithfully rather than risk denying it through an exclusive hope for a miracle.

Praying for Miracles

Because Jesus healed and because healings still occur, Christians naturally pray for miracles. As Richard expressed in chapter 3, even after being told his condition was incurable, "Why not me?" Seeking a miracle can ease anxiety and give courage in the face of fear. If the crumbs from the King's table fall to one poor sinner, why not Richard or you or me?

These longings fuel prayers for miraculous intervention in Jesus's name. The sick pray. Family members pray, sometimes for the first time in years. Moved by love, church communities often surround the ill with meals, visits, prayer chains, and heartfelt pleading that God would overturn a doctor's verdict. Jesus himself said, "If you have faith like a grain of mustard seed, . . . nothing will be impossible for you" (Matt. 17:20). Some Christians begin to think that if enough people pray hard enough, God will be compelled to respond. While this impulse is often energized by love and hope, it subtly misunderstands prayer as a matter of numbers pressing a reluctant or distant judge. This misses how God is a loving Father whose will is always for our good and our salvation.

The remarkable advances of medicine can at times lead the faithful to look for miracles through medical means. When Arthur, Richard, and Helen were told by their doctors that there was nothing more medicine could do, they resisted and clung to the hope that medicine would serve as the instrument for a miracle. This tendency is reinforced by the inherent uncertainty of medicine, especially in prognostication. As a Texan pastor said in one of our interviews regarding his Hispanic congregation, "I constantly hear stories from them to whom doctors said were going to die in two, three, four months. But then they are still alive ten or fifteen years later." Physicians may, at times, express undue certainty about the future for a patient only to be proven wrong. Such misjudgments can result in distrust of medical expertise regarding prognosis and fuel determination to keep hoping for a miracle, even with a dim prognosis.

The church itself can also unintentionally encourage an imbalanced focus on miracles through misunderstandings about God's healing. Scripture calls believers to pray in faith: "The prayer of faith will save the one who is sick" (James 5:15). Yet there is a fine line between faithful prayer and presumption. Claiming certainty about an outcome before it occurs can risk treating God as if he were obligated to act. As an Irish Catholic priest told us, "God is not your secretary. God is not your genie lamp." The priest then urged prayer shaped by Mary's words: "Let it be to me according to your word" (Luke 1:38).

Some in the prosperity gospel teach that it is *always* God's will to heal physical illness. Kenneth Hagin writes, "One giant step towards receiving healing for your physical body is to settle the issue that healing is the will of God for you."[11] Hagin presents disease as belonging solely to the enemy and physical healing as the believer's rightful inheritance. Yet Scripture offers a more complex witness. Paul pleaded three times for healing, only to hear, "My grace is enough for you" (2 Cor. 12:9 NCV). Lazarus was raised but later died again. Even Hagin himself eventually died. While God opposes illness and death, he permits their presence until Christ finally destroys death itself (1 Cor. 15:26; Rev. 20:14). Faith, therefore, should not presume how God intends to heal. Sometimes healing is physical. At other times it is emotional, relational, or spiritual. This was the healing Uncle Mike experienced. As one African Methodist Episcopal pastor told us, "Death itself may be the cure to what ails you."

As Christians pray for miracles, they must also recognize the danger of fostering false hope in a culture of death denial. In one study, 78 percent of terminally ill cancer patients affirmed belief in the possibility of a miracle. At a time of great vulnerability, false hope—however well-intentioned—can cause spiritual harm to ill persons and their loved ones. It is often easier for a spiritual leader to speak optimistically about possibilities for miraculous physical healing rather than acknowledge painful realities. This is especially the case when the seriously ill hold on to a miracle as a religiously justified way to avoid the reality of a poor prognosis.

In one instance, after praying in the hospital room of a congregant with a life-threatening infection, a pastor announced in a confident tone, "I sense that the Spirit has heard our prayer and that good things are coming." In another situation, after much prayer and medical treatment, a person with a serious heart condition experienced a degree of recovery for a time. And during the period of remission, fellow congregants claimed a miraculous cure had taken place, only for the person to die of their disease two months later. In the first scenario, the pastor could have taken care to emphasize that the "good things coming" could be physical or relational or spiritual healing. In regard to the second scenario, congregants could still praise God for the gift of healing but not presume the amount of time. Lois herself interpreted her first set of imaging scans after her kidney surgery in June 2021—which showed no evidence of cancer—as a miraculous cure from God. Supporting church members shared praises to God for the gift of this news but purposefully did not echo the language of a miraculous healing. Notably, only a few months later, Lois's next scans showed metastases.

Physical healing is a good we as Christians are encouraged to seek out and pray for (James 5:14–15), but it should never be the final goal. Rather, it is but an instrument for greater, enduring purposes that speak of God's kingdom and glory. But all too commonly the physical goal of healing is all that is hoped for, not the deeper forms of healing that are eternal. That was the healing experienced by Uncle Mike—a healing far more powerful and enduring than if he had jumped off his ICU bed and walked out the hospital doors.

Entering a hospital room and boldly praying for a healing miracle can set up the vulnerable for spiritual disillusionment. As one hospital chaplain explained to us, the risk of giving false hope for a miracle is that "it puts God on trial." Hospital chaplains are especially well-attuned to navigate complex, and often hidden, psychological dynamics intertwined with spirituality. Community clergy would do well to learn from and partner with local hospital chaplains.[12]

When the miracle doesn't come and illness advances, the person can wonder why God has abandoned them. That said, when a church leader, fellow congregant, or loved one is called upon to pray for a miracle, such a prayer of faith can and should be sincerely offered. However, together with prayers for healing should always be the aim to ask for more enduring forms of spiritual growth, such as addressing fears. Not uncommonly, underneath the request for a miracle are unaddressed fears. The shepherding task is both to earnestly ask God for a healing miracle and to seek spiritual growth. This includes addressing the patient's fears in a manner that brings hope in God regardless of the outcome of the illness.

Addressing Fears

When Christians cling to the hope of a miracle in the face of serious illness, we must also be mindful of the unconscious anxiety and fear that may lie beneath the surface. When we are accompanying someone through serious illness, or experiencing serious illness ourselves, it can be helpful to invite honest reflection on these fears by asking thoughtful questions and listening attentively for unacknowledged fears.

Consider questions like

- "As you think about the future, have you been feeling any fear?"
- "How do you cope, especially in moments that feel overwhelming?"
- "If a miracle does not come, what other ways might God help that could give you peace or a sense of readiness for what comes next?"

One powerful way to normalize the experience of fear is to contemplate the example of Jesus before his own death. As he fervently prayed in Gethsemane, Jesus recognized it was not the Father's will to grant a miracle of rescue from death. In response, he was "in agony" (Luke 22:44). His disciples, unable to face their own sorrow, fell asleep (v. 45). Jesus, the Son of God, though he did not have fear, experienced deep distress and anguish as death approached. If Jesus, the Son of God, though he did not have fear, experienced deep distress and anguish as death approached, then surely there is no shame in acknowledging our own distress and fears.

In this context, we should encourage prayer—not in denial of fear, but in its midst—just as Christ intensely prayed. Jesus asked for the miracle: "Father, if you are willing, remove this cup from me" (v. 42). But he also surrendered to the Father's will: "Nevertheless, not my will, but yours, be done" (v. 42). We, too, can plead passionately for healing, while also accepting that God's plan may unfold differently. In the practice of intense, honest prayer, fears often rise to the surface. It is through prayer that God provides strength, sometimes through a message, sometimes through a messenger (v. 43).

A second way to address the fear of death is to nurture hope for the life to come. When the thief on the cross realized the true nature of Jesus, he humbled himself by acknowledging Jesus's identity and his own sinfulness (Luke 23:41). The thief then humbled himself further by asking Christ to "remember me when you come into your kingdom" (v. 42). This was a remarkable statement of faith, since the thief could see that Jesus was himself dying.

Jesus responded, "Truly, I say to you, today you will be with me in paradise" (v. 43). The promise of "today" was immediate: "sharing an afterlife *that very day* with Jesus himself."[13] Rather than affirming the thief's request to be in the kingdom in some ambiguous future time, Jesus's promise was that on that very day the thief would join him "in paradise." Originally an ancient Persian idea of a garden, paradise as understood by the Jews is a gloriously restored garden of Eden, which righteous souls enter upon death. This is the "garden of God" (Ezek. 31:8), where there is joy, gladness, and song (Isa. 51:3). In Christ, the dead immediately enter a new experience aptly described by St. Augustine: "On that day we shall rest and see, see and love, love and praise—for this is to be the end without the end of all our living, that Kingdom without end, the real goal of our present life."[14]

When we are moved to pray for a miracle during serious illness, whether for someone else or for ourselves, we must soberly consider the possible presence of fear and of death denial. Jesus's promise to the thief on the cross of immediate entrance into paradise reveals a better miracle (Luke 23:43). To enter paradise is a far greater marvel than physical healing because it is a permanent healing of the soul. When promises about heaven are clearly held before the suffering person, fear often loosens and hope flourishes even in the face of death. Uncle Mike was a clear example of this. Christians rightly affirm that God can heal the body at any time he chooses. Yet in spiritual care, it is a mistake to underemphasize salvation as the greatest miracle God gives. We should pray and hope for physical healing, while nurturing within others and ourselves a recognition of the wondrous reality of far greater forms of healing. Jesus could have offered the thief a brief escape from death, but instead God answered the deepest cry for a miracle by granting him enduring paradise—an infinitely greater gift.

One meaningful way to grow hope despite illness is to invite ourselves and those we care for to imagine the paradise of heaven. Though we only "see through a glass, darkly" (1 Cor. 13:12 KJV), many find immense peace by envisioning what awaits us when we die in Christ.

Ask questions like

- "What do you think it might be like when you enter God's heaven?"

- "Who are you looking forward to seeing again—or meeting for the first time?"
- "What would you like to ask God when you see him face-to-face?"

This kind of hopeful imagination can help release fear of the unknown and awaken a sense of anticipation, peaceful comfort, and joy.

A third way to confront fear of death is to inquire about any final acts of love the person may wish to offer prior to death. You might gently ask questions like

- "Is there something loving in your heart that still needs to be said or done before your time in this life ends?"
- "Is there someone who keeps coming to mind to whom perhaps you are to impart a word of encouragement or help?"

Scripture says, "There is no fear in love. But perfect love drives out fear" (1 John 4:18 NIV). Fear unchecked leads to death denial. In the face of fear, we must fix our eyes on God's love manifest in Christ's death for our sin and his promise of the eternal life to come. This is the only reality that overcomes the fear of death, enabling us to, in Christ, triumphantly declare, "O death, where is your sting?" (1 Cor. 15:55). Pondering centrally in our hearts the truth of our eternal life in Christ, together with prayerful consideration of loving, meaningful, and heartfelt final earthly actions, stirs courage and restores a sense of God's presence and purpose in dying.

Healing Comes in Many Forms

Christians facing illness and those providing spiritual care to them should respond with faith when called to pray for a miracle. At the same time, we must remember that God brings healing and wholeness in many forms, even when the body is not restored. As Uncle Mike lay on his deathbed, after weeks of deep fear, a simple and sincere prayer of repentance brought a profound change. His fear melted, and peace took its place. Just before he was sedated to never awake, he again said, this time to his children, "I feel peace." There was no physical healing, but a real miracle occurred that day.

In caring for others and in journeying through illness ourselves, we are called upon to follow the example of Jesus—both in Gethsemane, where he surrendered to the Father's will, and in his promise of paradise, which quiets fear and gives lasting hope. By doing this, we move toward a more enduring conception of healing that reaches far beyond physical illness and leads to a deeper peace found in knowing God and trusting in his salvation.

Seven

Struggle and Longing

After this, Jesus, knowing that all was now finished, said (to fulfill the Scripture), "I thirst." A jar full of sour wine stood there, so they put a sponge full of the sour wine on a hyssop branch and held it to his mouth.

John 19:28–29

What was really needed was a fundamental change in our attitude toward life. We had to learn ourselves and, furthermore, we had to teach the despairing men, that it did not really matter what we expected from life, but rather what life expected from us. We needed to stop asking about the meaning of life, and instead to think of ourselves as those who were being questioned by life—daily and hourly. Our answer must consist, not in talk and meditation, but in right action and in right conduct. Life ultimately means taking the responsibility to find the right answer to its problems and to fulfill the tasks which it constantly sets for each individual.

Victor Frankl

Those who care for patients with advanced dementia know for a fact that singing is one of the last remaining ways that people with

> advanced Alzheimer's can participate in the life of a community. . . . The community is forced to take a breath together, and to match their breath and their voices to one another. It joins the community together, and it's something beautiful to do for someone who's just beyond your reach.
>
> Lydia Dugdale

THE FIRST TIME we visited Lois together was a few months after her kidney removal surgery and soon after the discovery of metastatic spread. She met us at her apartment in Winthrop, Massachusetts. Her building was situated on the Boston Harbor. The wind was strong that day, blowing in stiff gusts off the water. Dark clouds were forming on the horizon. A rainstorm would hit during our visit. But here and there, beams of light broke through, shining within patches of blue.

Lois had grown up in Winthrop. She had always loved the ocean. To her, it was full of mystery and power. It brought life and excitement. When she was a child, her house had looked out over a small harbor inlet. Now, from the eleventh floor of her apartment building, she could smell the salty air and feel the breeze off the sea.

Lois was starting to think about death. She didn't know it yet, but she had less than a year to live. Still, you could tell the thought was on her mind. She told us she wanted her ashes to be spread in Boston Harbor, just as she had done for her father. She spoke about him with warmth; he had been the perfect dad.

Later, we learned more. As a child, Lois was doted on by her mother and father, but as she grew into a young woman, her father in particular was not easy to please. He was a gruff man—a fisherman with a tough shell who didn't show love easily. She longed to be close to him as she was when she was a girl, but she never felt she was enough. He often criticized her, including her love for art and her decision to get an art degree. He disapproved of the man she fell in love with in her twenties and ultimately married. His disapproval only deepened when they divorced a few years later. His criticisms landed deep within her.

This longing and distance also shaped how Lois saw God. She believed in God and even wanted to be close to him. But God felt far away. He was hard to understand. Lois had tender emotions. She was easily hurt and sensitive to anything that felt like rejection. Over time, she started to keep her distance from God. She thought he was harsh. He was like the ocean—beautiful, but powerful and unpredictable. She could admire him from her balcony, but it felt safer to keep a distance.

During her midlife years, Lois spread her father's ashes in the harbor. After that, she seemed to find peace about their relationship. She rarely spoke of his rough side again. We only learned about it after her death, from friends who had known her since childhood. We were shocked to learn how her relationship with her dad was chaotic for many years, so different from her own accounting to us.

In those midlife years, Lois found a form of peace with God. Not closeness. It was more like a truce. Lois in her relationship to God was friendly but distant. There was no storm but no spiritual intimacy either.

Now, later in life, her diagnosis came. The peace she had known began to break apart. The quiet distance between her and God felt less safe. Old questions of rejection and abandonment came swirling back.

"Why is God against me?" she asked.

"What did I do to deserve this? Is God punishing me for my sins?"

"Why can't he just let me live in peace?"

The storm returned. The God she had kept at a safe distance was now near. This profoundly frightened her. To Lois, God felt again like her father and like the sea she yearned for and yet feared. Strong. Beautiful. But deeply troubling. Sometimes harsh. Lois longed for a closer relationship, but God felt distant and unsafe.

Spiritual Struggle

Lois's experience is far from unique. Her story reveals a common spiritual pattern: Many people avoid unresolved questions about God during times of health, opting instead to live in a state of suspended belief—anchored in the harbor, neither securely docked nor willing to venture deeper. But serious illness is like a sudden storm that blows the ship unwillingly near jagged rocks. When pushed against the breakers, the soul is forced to confront what it once avoided. The need for what is truly real becomes urgent and inescapable.

Struggle with God is widespread, cutting across religions, cultures, and age groups, and experienced by those who are very religious, spiritual but not religious, or even atheistic.[1] Among 17,000 Americans, 32 percent reported struggling with the divine and 43 percent sought ultimate meaning.[2]

Spiritual struggles tend to increase as illness becomes more severe. Among cancer survivors, studies show that between 15 and 48 percent report experiencing spiritual struggle.[3] As sick persons come closer to facing their own mortality, questions about their relationship with God often become more urgent. In a national survey of 1,885 seriously ill patients and caregivers, the two highest ranked needs out of forty-four identified were pain control and finding peace with God.[4] Similarly, in a multisite survey of 331 patients with advanced cancer receiving palliative care, 66 percent reported some level of spiritual struggle, and 20 percent reported moderate to high levels of struggle in at least one area.[5]

Our own study conducted at four Boston-area hospitals found that 86 percent of cancer patients endorsed some degree of spiritual concerns, including 58 percent reporting at least one type of difficult spiritual struggle.[6] Specific kinds included the following:

- 20 percent were doubting the existence of God
- 25 percent were angry toward God
- 29 percent felt abandoned by God
- 22 percent thought the cancer was God's punishment for sin or lack of devotion
- 25 percent questioned God's personal love

At the same time, most were also spiritually seeking:

- 54 percent said they were seeking a closer connection with God
- 48 percent were thinking about being forgiven or forgiving others
- 54 percent were thinking about meaning in life or seeking meaning in their cancer

Notably, in this study and others, younger patients facing serious illness often have more unresolved spiritual struggles. Furthermore, even among those who do not identify as religious, spiritual needs are common.[7] This is evident in the case of Margaret, a thirty-nine-year-old never-married woman with metastatic colorectal cancer.[8] She was too sick to continue working as an attorney in immigration law. When we first interviewed her, she matter-of-factly stated that spiritual care was irrelevant to her. "I am not spiritual or religious," she told us. If we had not asked follow-up questions, her spiritual pain would have remained under the surface.

As our interview progressed, Margaret revealed a more complex picture. She shared that she had been raised Roman Catholic, though she no longer attended services and was uncertain about her current beliefs. Despite her initial disavowal of spirituality, she admitted feeling punished by God and questioning God's power. She also spoke of asking for forgiveness for her sins and seeking strength from God. She was angry toward God and full of doubt on what to believe about spiritual realities.

Margaret's story illustrates the phenomenon of spiritual ambivalence. Providing legal support to refugees gave her life purpose. Apart from this, and in a place of struggle with God, despair had set in. She was fighting her disease and wrestling with God. We asked if she would like to speak with a chaplain, but she declined. Margaret's soul was longing for the eternal, but she resisted it at the same time.

"I Thirst"

Jesus's fifth word from the cross, the Greek *dipsaō*—translated "I thirst" (John 19:28)—expresses a deep spiritual longing. On the simplest level, he is expressing real physical suffering. His body is in agony, his mouth is dry, and breathing is difficult. Medically, as a person is dying, dehydration and reduced saliva cause the mouth and tongue to become dry and thick. Swallowing and breathing are uncomfortable. Small doses of water, often given today through ice chips, are used to moisten the mouth and bring relief. In this moment, Jesus fully shares in the weakness and vulnerability of human life.

But more is happening than physical thirst alone. When Jesus says, "I thirst," he also reveals a deeper emptiness that belongs to our human condition. Nothing in this world can fully satisfy the soul. All of life's temporal comforts fall short. This is especially striking in the Gospel of John, where Jesus told the Samaritan woman that whoever drinks physical water will only thirst again, whereas those who drink the water he gives will never thirst again

(John 4:14). The one who quenches all thirst now enters fully into our longing. At the same time, his words echo the cry of the psalms, a soul thirsting for God in a dry and weary land (Ps. 42:1). In this sense, "I thirst" is both a word of spiritual struggle and a word of longing: struggle because the Father's felt distance causes affliction and longing as he, turning away from every false source of satisfaction, desires only the living God. Only God is the true fulfillment of his longing.

From Struggle to Disillusionment

When the soul experiences such thirst and the stripping away of this life in serious illness, it can lead, such as in the case of Margaret, to internal collapse. Viktor Frankl tragically illustrates this in *Man's Search for Meaning*, as he recounts surviving the Holocaust and life in the Auschwitz concentration camp.[9] Frankl observed that some prisoners, when overtaken by hopelessness, ceased to respond to their surroundings. They no longer reacted to Nazi beatings, threats, or commands. Once this mental collapse set in, they typically died within days. It was a deeper form of death, an erasure of the will to live even before the body succumbed.

Frankl also warns against the danger of false hope. Some survivors clung to a hope that they would be reunited with their families after liberation, only to discover that their loved ones had perished. This led many into despair and aimlessness, despite their earlier resilience. Frankl describes such individuals as drifting like ships without a rudder. Alive but unanchored. When we seek to satisfy the thirst of the soul with temporal things, no matter how good, we are bound for disillusionment.

In contrast, spiritual struggle indicates that the soul is longing for something sure and unshakable. Illness strips away the illusion that the things of this life can satisfy. For this reason, engaging spiritual struggle in relationship with God is central to the experience of illness and to the care of the sick. The soul is admitting that it may have been misled by false hopes. Any prior ambivalence toward or dismissal of God must now be reconsidered as the soul longs for something greater. The calling, upon those enduring the trial of illness and those providing spiritual care to them, is to move toward the sustenance found in the Living Water while crying out, "I thirst."

The Struggle of Dementia

One disease that often leads to such disillusionment is dementia. Dementia is a progressive, incurable neurocognitive disorder resulting in deterioration of memory, reasoning, and executive function. A death-denying culture dreads dementia because it slowly and publicly reveals the loss of control, independence, and self-defined identity—all deeply held cultural values. Both people living with dementia and their caregivers struggle with God, face isolation, and are at risk for despair.[10]

Irene is an eighty-year-old woman with a strong Christian faith who had been dealing with memory issues for some years, but she recently received a formal diagnosis of Alzheimer's. Sitting in her favorite chair, she spoke slowly, sometimes having difficulty with her words. She repeatedly reminded herself that she had five children, saying it out loud to hold on to something steady. Pastor Brian came to visit Irene at the request of her daughter. Irene shared how she had seen the devastation of dementia in her extended family and watched loved ones lose their independence and dignity. She dreaded this future.

At one point, she said quietly, "I feel like I'm losing who I am."

Pastor Brian responded, "You are not lost to God or to us. You are known and loved. We will go with you through this." Her fear was met with presence.

In contrast to a cultural narrative of loss, Christians believe that a person's worth does not rest on memory or ability but on being known and loved by God. Dementia does not undo faith or one's belonging to the body of Christ. God does not forget his children (Isa. 44:21). As Swinton has argued, the church upholds people with dementia by trusting that they are already held in the faithful memory of God.[11]

Irene voiced this struggle: "How will I have faith if I cannot even remember who God is?"

Pastor Brian pondered this and then answered, "Even if your faith no longer looks or sounds the way it used to, God remains faithful and will never forget you. We will find ways so that you can continue to worship with us."

This response affirmed that faith is not something a person must hold alone, nor is faith only cognitive.[12] Faith is shared in the body of Christ, and communities carry individuals.

People living with early-stage dementia often enter a terrifying experience of knowing they are losing parts of themselves. They fear becoming a burden and live with a socially stigmatized illness. When Irene voiced her fear of becoming a burden for her family, Pastor Brian replied, "Your life is not a burden to God or to this community. None of us want this future for you, but if this is what God is permitting, then we can trust the Lord hears the cry of our souls. Good will somehow come from this evil." He then offered a concrete act of care. He suggested that someone from the church could come to her home to listen to her story and record her testimony. They could record her faith, her memories, her prayers, and anything she wanted her family to hear. These recordings could be played back anytime, allowing her to hear her own story even on days when her memory failed.

Whereas individuals falter, Christian community can hold suffering and memory despite the struggle. When dementia takes personal memory, the community carries it, holding the person's story and sharing in suffering even as the individual may stumble.[13]

Family caregivers also suffer deeply because of dementia. This is a form of moral suffering, as Harvard psychiatrist Arthur Kleinman described during his years of caring for his spouse afflicted with dementia.[14] Caregiving is frequently private, exhausting, and lonely. It involves grief without closure or reciprocity, as the person the caregiver loves slowly changes. This ongoing loss can lead to despair.

The moral suffering of caregivers can be shared within a spiritual community. Rather than turning away, the church can step forward. Through visitation and community support, meaning can be found in shared action. During Sunday services, church leaders should learn names and stories of those who are struggling with memory loss and practice simple hospitality. When Irene wandered off and became lost after leaving for the bathroom during worship, an attentive church leader noticed her confusion. The lay leader smiled, offered a hand, and said, "Hello, Irene. I'm so glad to see you. May I walk you back to your seat?"

Some churches have developed dementia-focused ministries by shaping services around familiar hymns, simple prayers, and brief sermons. Others bring worship services with familiar music into assisted living facilities, offering comfort to both residents and staff. Support groups gather caregivers online to share their stories and provide mutual encouragement. Pastoral visitation should continue even as dementia progresses. It may include listening to Scripture on audio, playing sacred music, or bringing familiar religious objects as gentle reminders of faith. During home visits, singing hymns together can be especially meaningful, since musical memory is often preserved even when other memories fade. When prayer becomes difficult, a pastor might say, "Let me pray with you. God hears us even when words are hard to find."

In the ongoing struggle, when the loss of memory and abilities places the soul at risk of despair, spiritual communities have an opportunity to form what Kleinman calls a bond of emotion and meaning.[15] We would also suggest that when we share in the suffering person's thirst for the eternal, a spiritual bond is formed. And though difficult, this bond brings hidden fruits. It forces the healthy to admit that nothing in this life can satisfy while it manifests deepening forms of meaning and love in Christ. For communities willing to share in this burden, the promise of transformation and hope shines bright.

Job's Turmoil

The story of Job illustrates the spiritual struggle that illness can provoke. Unlike Lois or Margaret, Job began in deep friendship with God (Job 29:2–5). But when disaster struck—loss of health, family, and livelihood—Job's theology unraveled. He accused God of being unjust (21:30–31), cruel (16:9–14), and silent (9:11). He believed God had become his enemy (19:11), though he could find no justified reason for divine disapproval (23:6–7).

Job's friends, meant to be his comforters, turned into accusers. They insisted that Job's suffering must be punishment for hidden sin. Their rigid theology couldn't accommodate divine mystery. In contrast, the book of Job invites readers to wrestle with complexity. It questions the simplistic equation of suffering equals sin.

Scripture affirms that while sin causes suffering (Gen. 3), not all suffering results from sin. Job, declared "blameless and upright" by God (Job 2:3), suffered not because of wrongdoing but for reasons beyond his understanding. Jesus echoed this in John 9:2–3, rejecting the disciples' assumption that a man's blindness was due to punishment.

This mistake, believing suffering is always earned, comforts some because it offers control and a reason for suffering. But it is false. Sometimes, suffering arrives not in judgment but as an invitation. Job's suffering becomes a cosmic testimony. God permits the trial because he trusts Job's love. More deeply, God believes in grace's power to uphold the human heart.

"Shall we accept good from God, and not trouble?" (Job 2:10 NIV). This question, spoken by Job in the midst of profound loss, gets to the heart of the matter: Can I trust God when the gifts are gone? Job's suffering came not because he had sinned but ironically because he loved and respected God. And in a heavenly courtroom far beyond Job's knowledge, Satan had issued a challenge: "Does Job fear God for nothing?" (1:9 NIV). The accusation was not just about Job. It was an indictment of humanity and a defamation of God's worth. The implication of Satan's question was simple: Humans only love God for divine blessings. Remove the gifts, and they will curse him. So God permitted Satan to strike Job but not to destroy him.

Job is never told the reason for his suffering. And that's essential. Had God explained everything, Job might have endured with ulterior motives. But silence preserved the purity of Job's faith. The patience of Job, despite the silence of God, disproved Satan's allegations.

This is the invitation to all who suffer without knowing why: When the tide of illness rises and the crushing rocks are close, we can trust the God who holds the ocean in his hands. As God eventually responds later in the book of Job, not with answers but with questions of his own, the Lord asserts not only his sovereignty but also his divine wisdom. He reminds Job, and us, that though the world is more intricate than we can fathom, it still rests in the hands of a good God.

Not always but sometimes, God's Spirit lets us glimpse behind the curtain. The book of Job, in its full arc, suggests something profound: Innocent suffering is the very tool God uses to redeem. From the first animal sacrificed in Genesis to cover Adam and

Eve, to the lambs offered under Mosaic law, and finally to Jesus Christ—the Lamb of God—Scripture paints a consistent picture: The innocent sufferer mysteriously brings healing and restoration to others.

Job's suffering mirrors this redemptive arc. His pain silences Satan. His prayers reconcile his friends to God. His endurance becomes a testimony through the ages. And ultimately, Job points us to Christ. Jesus, the true Innocent Sufferer, who bore the weight of sin not his own, was misunderstood, accused, abandoned, and crucified. Yet in his suffering, redemption was gifted to the world. Likewise, when we face serious illness, we are being drawn into that same cosmic mystery. The soul is forced to acknowledge false hopes, face despair, and experience dissatisfaction and longing. It is a spiritual thirst encountered by the seriously ill and those around them.

Facing Our Emptiness

Jesus's words "I thirst" echo the longing in Psalm 69: "I looked for sympathy, but there was none, for comforters, but I found none" (v. 20 NIV). This cry reveals his vulnerability and need. Instead of care, Jesus was given a bitter drink. It was a cruel response from those who chose judgment rather than compassion.

The vinegar Jesus received recalls what Job endured. Job called his friends "miserable comforters" (16:2) and "worthless physicians" (13:4). They failed to comfort him and instead added to his suffering. A similar response appears in the Gospels when the Pharisees judged the man born blind. These responses are not limited to the past. Even today, we face the same choice when encountering serious illness. We can offer vinegar, or we can offer water.

Making this choice requires caregivers to face their own emptiness. We can offer vinegar to the sick when our own souls are unsettled and unexamined. Serious illness confronts the healthy with questions we would often rather avoid. It exposes the limits of comfort found in circumstances, success, or possessions. The sick remind us that true life, meaning, and fulfillment are found in God alone. We accompany the sick most faithfully when we recognize our own deep thirst and bring it honestly before God. If we judge like Job's counselors, mock suffering like the soldiers at the cross, or avoid the seriously ill altogether, many of us actually avoid our own vulnerability. The sick remind us that we, too, cry out, "I thirst."

Spiritual healing for both the sick and their caregivers requires engaging suffering directly. It means facing spiritual struggle rather than escaping it. Healing does not come by avoiding pain but by wrestling with God. In that struggle, the soul begins to drink from what is eternal.

Frankl describes this kind of struggle in *Man's Search for Meaning*. Stripped of identity and dignity in Auschwitz, he found that even extreme suffering could not destroy his deepest self or separate him from ultimate meaning. While digging a trench in the snow of Bavaria, exhausted and near despair, his soul wrestled with the question of whether there was any reason for his suffering and slow dying. As a guard insulted him and demanded more work, Frankl noticed a light shining from a distant farmhouse in the early morning gray. In that moment, words came to his mind: "The light shines in the darkness." He experienced this not as a momentary thought but as a transcendent voice answering the cry of his soul. The Spirit's response was a clear and unmistakable yes. Even in misery and fear, he discovered meaning. This encounter later shaped Frankl's work of helping others endure suffering without losing dignity or purpose.

The apostle Paul describes a similar path in Romans 5:3–5, where suffering produces endurance, endurance forms character, and character gives rise to hope. Paul does not praise suffering itself. Instead, he shows how God works within it to transform the soul. This transformation applies both to those who are seriously ill and to those who care for them. Arthur Kleinman reflects on his years caring for his wife, Joan, during her dementia as a long endurance. Through it, he writes that he "emerged remade" and morally formed by suffering in ways that led to deep hope.[16] Whether in concentration camps, dementia, or the process of dying, Paul points to the same truth. Even in the most dehumanizing conditions, our thirst can be quenched by the eternal.

Illness and caregiving press us to ask a difficult question: Who am I when everything else is taken away? Like metal refined by fire, character formed through adversity becomes the place where our deepest longings are clarified. This was true for Job, for Paul, and most fully for Jesus. It is also seen in the lives of Viktor, Irene, and Lois. As the soul releases what cannot sustain it, it begins to long for what is eternal.

Lois Comes Home

Lois had been anxious for months. She moved from hospitals to rehab centers and could not return to her apartment. Because of restrictions, visitors were limited, and the fear that she would end up in a nursing home and die alone stayed with her constantly. As I (Tracy) look back now, I can see that long before the crisis came fully into view, God had already begun working quietly in me to reveal that we were called to bring Lois into our home.

For some time before Lois was faced with the possibility of going to a nursing home to die, the thought had come to me more than once. I knew how fearful she was of being alone, and I recognized that it could very well end that way for her. More than once I found myself thinking, almost to my surprise, that maybe we should take her into our home. I did not say it out loud at first. I carried it silently, praying about it, trying to understand whether it was simply concern or something the Spirit was asking me to do. Only later did I learn that Michael had been wondering the same thing.

At first, when Lois was accepted into inpatient hospice, it seemed that the question had been resolved—this was a setting where she could have visitors and where there was adequate attention to her complex symptoms. She was quite sick, and we truly believed she would die within a few weeks of arriving at the inpatient hospice facility. But then Lois began to improve, and once she improved, she no longer qualified to remain in inpatient hospice. Suddenly, the question returned.

When it became clear that Lois's only care option was to go to a skilled nursing facility, Michael and I finally talked openly with one another. In that conversation, we realized we both had been grappling with the same question. We committed the decision to prayer and had conversations with our teenage children. In response, we saw how God was opening the door to have Lois in our home and taking care of every detail to make it possible. For example, we knew a woman named Mary who was studying to become a nurse and needed clinical experience. She enthusiastically accepted the job of being a nursing aid to Lois. Mary would tend to Lois during the day, and then Michael and I would take over in the evenings and on weekends. With many forms of confirmation, we accepted taking Lois into our home as God's calling for us.

When Lois learned she could no longer remain at the inpatient hospice facility, she panicked. Lois called everyone she knew for help and desperately appealed to the hospice manager for an exception. The thought of moving into an isolated nursing home completely overwhelmed her. It was in the middle of that crisis when I called Lois.

"Lois, I want to ask you something. Michael and I have been praying about this for some time, and we believe God wants us to invite you to come into our home—be a part of our family—and receive hospice care with us. Would you want to do this?"

There was a long silence, and then she let out one of her unmistakable sounds of exuberance, half laugh and half cry. "Oh, Tracy. Oh, you have no idea," she exclaimed. "I cannot believe it! Yes. Yes! Thank you. I cannot tell you how happy this makes me. What an answer to prayer."

Two days later, she arrived by ambulance on a cold February afternoon. She was fragile and uncertain. As she was carried up the stairs and saw her room for the first time, I remember her reaction clearly. "Oh my God, this room is incredible. I can't believe I'm here with you. Thank you, God. Thank you, Tracy. Thank you, Michael."

Sunlight filled the room and fell across a bouquet of fresh flowers that had just been given by someone from the church. For entirely unrelated reasons, the room had been freshly painted and furnished, and the curtains we had ordered six months earlier were installed as the final touch just the day before. Even though we had not known until forty-eight hours earlier that Lois would be coming, the room was ready. The Spirit had been preparing both the space and our hearts to welcome Lois.

What we did not know then was that the few weeks of care I had anticipated would become six months. Six months of struggle, longing, and unexpected transformation for Lois and for all of us who walked with her.

Eight

Seeking Life, Accepting Death

For everything there is a season, and a time for every matter under heaven:

> a time to be born, and a time to die.

Ecclesiastes 3:1–2

When Jesus had received the sour wine, he said, "It is finished," and he bowed his head and gave up his spirit.

John 19:30

I have seen people who have come out of diseases saying, "This ain't my time to die. I got too much going on." And they didn't die. One guy survived AIDS. He said, "I got too much going. I don't sense that dying is what God wants for me to do." There is God's timing and there is also the sovereignty of God. Sometimes it is hard to tell. I think there is a mystery in it.

Pastor, Chicago

THROUGH SPIRITUAL STRUGGLE, our desire for life can shift to a deeper longing for God. As one makes this internal shift in the face of death, the ability to let go emerges. Scripture gives us both a command to choose life and a reminder that death is not the end. In the Christian life, we are called to hold these two truths—seeking life and accepting death—in prayerful discernment.

Richard's Purpose

At forty-nine years old, Richard was not ready to die. And no one—not doctors, nurses, nor his own crumbling body—could convince him otherwise. As we read in chapter 3, Richard fired Dr. Patel as his doctor, refusing to accept the doctor's assessment that he should go home with hospice care. As sure as his faith in Christ, he believed a miracle would come.

He was a man with a purpose. A father, husband, and provider. "If I were an older guy," he once told a nurse, "I think I would have much less attachment to survival. But we each have a certain work to do on earth, and I need to finish mine." For Richard, that work was raising his daughters, especially the one with Down syndrome. Deep in his bones he knew that they needed him. And he would not, could not, abandon them.

Faith was never far from Richard's thoughts. His belief in God was not abstract. It was deeply woven into his hopes, identity, and decisions. He believed that healing was possible, maybe even imminent. "God will use whatever means at his disposal to effect a cure," he said more than once. From medicine to a miracle, all were in play. And as he reflected on the words of Jesus, about faith as small as a mustard seed moving mountains, he saw firsthand that Christ was a God who heard his prayers and had already done one miracle.

To many of his doctors, Richard was difficult. He challenged their recommendations, rejected timelines, and sneered at their prognosis. Some clinicians spoke behind his back that he was arrogant, combative. He didn't make it easy to see a father whose heart was aching to remain in this world for just a little longer to fulfill what he believed was his God-given responsibility as a father.

But one person understood.

Nurse Patrick had been by Richard's side for years. Roughly the same age and sharing the same denominational faith and passion for college hockey, Patrick saw in Richard not a difficult patient but a man holding tightly to his calling. Their relationship deepened after Richard confided about a moment in the ICU about a year earlier, when, intubated and on the brink of death, Richard had heard God speak: *It is not time for you yet*. Richard then recovered. The doctors had no explanation other than it was just one of those rare cases that defied prognosis. And from that point on, he believed—rather, he *knew*—he was supposed to live.

Patrick listened. He asked questions. He prayed with Richard. Sometimes in silence, sometimes aloud. Together they recited the Lord's Prayer, their combined voices bringing spiritual life into the halls of medicine.

But time and metastatic cancer continued their march. Cancer grew in his chest, pressing on his airways and his esophagus. Surgeons debated risky procedures. A family meeting was called in which the medical team outlined how they were "out of options" in treating the cancer and that hospice should be considered. Tensions boiled over as Richard lashed out. A father determined to provide for and protect his children was furious, cornered, terrified.

Choose Life

Most Christians believe that choosing life honors God, the giver of life. In one study, nearly 70 percent of seriously ill Christians agreed with the statement, "I accept every medical treatment because my faith says to do everything I can to stay alive."[1] This response reflects a sincere theological conviction that preserving life is a sacred duty, rooted in the belief that life itself is a divine gift. Scripture affirms this: "Truly, no ransom avails for one's life. . . . For the ransom of life is costly" (Ps. 49:7–8 NRSVA); we are urged to "choose life" (Deut. 30:19), commanded to "love your neighbor as yourself" (Matt. 22:39), and prohibited from taking life unjustly (Exod. 20:13). This loving reverence for life shapes not only how we think about the end of life but also how we view its beginning, including questions about elective abortion. In the Christian tradition, to preserve life at its beginning and end is to honor the Creator who gives every breath.

Christians' deep moral calling to affirm life is largely supported by the medical system. The default position of modern medicine is to preserve life. But of course, that drive to heal in medicine has its blind spots, as noted by one Boston pastor: "The medical field has a messianic complex: 'We can fix it all. You are sick? Don't worry. There is a solution for that too.'"

However, even when medicine recognizes its limits, as in Richard's case, many Christians have a deep impulse to fight the disease no matter what. Don, an older man recently informed of his terminal illness by his physician, told his thirty-year-old Texas pastor, "I have faith, and I want to live. I'm going down kicking and screaming. To hell with what they say."

His pastor knew that Don was at peace with God. He just loved life. So Pastor John said, "Whatever you decide I'm with you. You have my total support."

Like about 50 percent of people with metastatic cancer, Don pursued every possible medical option along with a range of complementary and alternative therapies.[2] While Don's physicians were more reserved about some of these therapies, Don found Pastor John's enthusiastic support to be encouraging.[3] In addition to a chemotherapy trial, he tried herbal remedies, juicing regimens, coffee enemas, and Ayurvedic breathing practices. Pastor John remained a steady prayer partner and personal encourager for nearly two years, until Don's death.

As Pastor John warmly reflected on Don's story, now twenty-five years later, he recalled: "I remember the day before he died, I went to go see him, and he could hardly talk the whole day. Don grabbed my hand and he told me, 'Thank you for being my friend and helping me in this process.' That is the last thing I heard from him. He did not speak again. But that is why I don't encourage people really to accept death. If they do, then fine. But if they have this thing to live, then I will encourage and support them."

Sometimes the impulse to fight comes from external pressures, driven by the family, once the doctors start suggesting that medicine has run its course. A number of pastors we interviewed indicated that family dynamics were often a strong driver toward aggressive medical therapies. One faith leader talked about an elderly congregant who had metastatic pancreatic cancer. "The family said that they had to do absolutely everything possible. Family members were not ready to lose their mother, their grandmother."

Churches can also make contributions to the motivation to pursue life at all costs.[4] As one California pastor serving a predominately Black congregation explained, it is the influence of faith, hope, and love. The community "thinks that if we can keep you going, keep praying and asking God. If we can get enough people to pray, then maybe we'll reach a threshold, and God will answer the prayer." It is also how the community expresses love to the sick. "We want to show that we love you by doing everything we possibly can to keep you with us. . . . We will fight for you, and we'll encourage you to do everything we can to keep you alive as long as possible as an expression of love."

And yet, in a national survey of US clergy, responses revealed a more nuanced theological posture. When asked if they agreed with the sentiment that faith demands every effort to sustain life, only 18 percent of clergy agreed "quite a bit or completely," while

46 percent disagreed entirely.[5] A majority (54 percent) of clergy saw at least some theological validity in this view. After taking into account factors like education level, the clergy most likely to show strong affirmation of faith requiring one to do everything to sustain life were Protestants from Pentecostal, Evangelical, and Historic Black Church communities. While there are important differences among Christians, a majority (including church leaders) tend to believe that all efforts must be pursued to sustain life. This shared belief can make it difficult to accept dying and to let go.

Letting Go

Affirming the sacredness of life must be balanced with accepting human finitude. As the apostle Peter recognized, "I know that the putting off of my body will be soon" (2 Pet. 1:14). Paul echoed this: "My life is being given as an offering to God, and the time has come for me to leave this life. I have fought the good fight, I have finished the race, I have kept the faith" (2 Tim. 4:6–7 NCV). Christian wisdom discerns when to let go.

Letting go of life is an act of surrender to our natural limits. While our instinct is to cling to life, our own and others', this drive can produce anxiety when life is threatened. As Jesus warned against hoarding possessions (Luke 12:13–21), he also called for trust in God's goodness as we recognize that life is outside our control (vv. 22–31). The pursuit of earthly things can be a way to avoid facing death; similarly, clinging to life may mask deeper fears.

Releasing our hold on this life is not simple. The struggle to hold on to life as an ultimate good is difficult to distinguish from a healthy emphasis on life's sacredness. But the remedy for such grasping, as theologian Allen Verhey suggested, is not a complete rejection of earthly things.[6] Such rejection would require denying the intrinsic value and goodness of these earthly gifts. For example, with Richard, his pursuit of life to remain a father to his children is hardly wrong. His desire to live for their sake is the fruit of his love for his children and his desire to secure their flourishing. These are undeniable goods worth pursuing.

Yet grasping for bodily life as if it is the only or ultimate good to be pursued, particularly in the face of dying, yields anxiety and despair. Jesus offered a way out of anxious grasping, even of life itself. He reminds us that this worldly life is brief and subject to relentless decay. We are admonished instead to put our treasure directly in God "where neither moth nor rust destroys and where thieves do not break in and steal" (Matt. 6:20). Furthermore, all in this life, including all good things such as children and the earthly role of a parent, must be surrendered, in trust, to God (Luke 12:20–21). Letting go does not mean we have stopped caring but that we are entrusting others to him who always cares. One person's death can be a catalyst for spiritual growth in another person. God uses sickness and death too. God cares, not just for birds and flowers but also for those we must let go of when we die (Luke 12:27–28). Thus, our energy should be spent on God's kingdom work, not holding on to the transitory goods of this life, including those we love and the important earthly callings we are temporarily given.

Letting go includes both lament and hope. Verhey explains, "Dying well requires that I do not cling to [family] anxiously as if I could expect them to save me from my mortality (or as if they have no hope without me), but it also requires that I do not discard them as distractions or prematurely alienate myself from them."[7] Letting go places these temporal goods into God's good hands. But the sadness that accompanies such surrender can and should be infused with hope. Jesus said, "Seek his kingdom, and these things will be given to you as well" (Luke 12:31 NIV). Hope in the kingdom is not an otherworldly focus. Verhey continues, "The good future of God, the kingdom of God, [is] the renewal and redemption of this world and these bodies."[8] In other words, one can lay down the good, including life itself, because God's promise is that it will return in due course but in an even better way.

Pursuing Cure or Comfort Care?

As we interviewed clergy around the United States, most argued that the decision to seek life versus letting go was a personal one.[9] A pastor in Chicago reflected: "It is about the person who is suffering. He is the one that decides if he wants to fight or wants to die. My goal as a pastor is whatever the patient decides."

Pastors from minority communities were especially attentive to protecting patient autonomy at the end of life. For many congregants who come from lower socioeconomic backgrounds, it would feel like another loss of dignity if the church was directive concerning medical decisions. These choices are understood as an expression of free will given by God to each person who is suffering, and the role of the church is to honor that choice rather than interfere. In a world where systems so often make decisions for those with fewer resources, many minority pastors emphasized that preserving a patient's right to choose may be one of the last ways that patient can claim dignity over their own life.

In the midst of serious illness, the sick often seek guidance from faith leaders and other congregants on how to approach this difficult choice. While honoring the patient's free-will decision is essential, it is equally important for pastors and church leaders to ask questions to help guide the exercise of free will through a maze of uncertainties. Noting this, one Baptist pastor said, "There is a difference between prolonging life and prolonging death. Prolonging life, when that is possible, is a good thing. But if it's simply to prolong this process of death, [then letting go] brings peace."

One factor informing a free-will decision is the medical prognosis and the degree of treatment burden. Catholic moral theology is a good guide for all Christians to consider. It helpfully calls on the sick to weigh the burden of receiving ongoing treatment. Will the treatment lead to greater pain and suffering? Will treatment increase or decrease quality of life? To what degree is the patient able to psychologically and physically tolerate additional treatments? Refusing burdensome treatments in the face of terminal illness is not willing one's own death but accepting its inevitability.[10] Pastoral and congregational caregivers do well not to impose answers but to ask questions that enable discernment.

There are also social factors that must be considered. What is the age of the patient? Does the sick person have children or other dependents? How ready is the family for the person's death? In many circumstances, there will be strong support to seek ongoing treatment when the patient is younger, has dependents, and when family members insist. Pastors often find themselves navigating these dynamics. During a focus group with pastors in Texas, several ministers agreed with a colleague who said, "I've been caught in the middle. Part of the family says we need to let him go, and other family members are furious, wanting to try everything. Dysfunctional family dynamics flower in circumstances like this." General pastoral wisdom in such cases is to invite everyone to pray and to focus on what the patient discerns is best. As a Presbyterian minister told us, "Everyone's opinion is valid. But in my experience the most important question we should all focus on is what does your mother [the patient] really want?"

Family meetings related to medical decisions are normally led by physicians and clinical teams. Ill persons and their families can consider inviting a trusted pastor or other faith leader for guidance and support during these meetings, or request a separate gathering.[11] In these moments, the pastoral role is to create space for family discernment, not choosing sides or forcing outcomes. Pastors can help bring family members together and facilitate conversation, often beginning with prayer and brief words from Scripture meant to invite love, patience, and peace. During a family meeting, several key issues and questions can be raised to both the ill person and their family members with the aim of clarifying everyone's understandings, hopes, and fears and of inviting the Holy Spirit to provide wisdom and clarity regarding decisions. At times, only family members are able to be present (e.g., when the sick person is sedated in the ICU). Such questions address

- Understanding the medical situation: Can you share what you understand the doctors to be saying right now, and what still feels unclear or confusing?
- Naming fears and hopes: What are you most afraid of in this moment, and what are you hoping for, even if it is hard to say out loud?
- Grounding the decision in faith: How does your faith shape the way you are thinking about this decision, and what do you believe God is asking of you right now?
- Honoring the patient's dignity: In light of your illness and your faith, what decision would most honor who you are, God's purposes for you, and your hopes? Or [when family answers for loved ones] what do you believe [the loved one] would want if they were making the decision for themselves? What would most honor them as a child of God and the life they have been given?

When Do You Let Go?

Upholding dignity is more straightforward when the ill person has the capacity to make his or her own medical decisions. As the sick deliberate benefits, burdens, and the needs and wishes of family, the primary focus for pastors and church members at the bedside is drawing the person to consider spiritual realities, including any unfinished spiritual work and/or spiritual issues that might be acting as roadblocks to letting go.

In the final hours of Jesus's life, he said "The hour has come" (Mark 14:41) and "It is finished" (John 19:30). In the original language, the word for "finished" means "completed" or "perfected." Jesus is saying that he has fulfilled all the work that has been given to him by the Father. On the cross, Christ bore all sin for the redemption of the world. Christ left nothing undone that had been asked of him by our heavenly Father. While only Jesus can fully say, "It is finished," this showcases an important discernment question between seeking life and accepting death. Jesus recognized that the time had come to let go because he had completed his life purpose.

It is important to know when you have been given a divine task that is still left undone. When King Hezekiah was told by the prophet Isaiah to get his house in order because his time was up, Hezekiah begged God for more time (2 Kings 20:1–6). Hezekiah's reason was that he was leaving his people in a place of disarray. Hezekiah was desperate for the sake of his love for Israel. In divine mystery, God surprisingly reversed the proclamation in response to prayer, giving Hezekiah fifteen more years to carry out unfinished business.

Such experiences still happen. One pastor from a predominately Haitian church had personally witnessed this dynamic. "I think there is a sense of calling and timing in the mind of God for people. I saw one lady in our church, almost like she shook off death nine times. I would go to the intensive care unit. Doctors said she was going to die. Her lung capacity is failing. All of a sudden, I get a call the next day saying, 'I don't know what happened. She turned around.'" There is a mystery to all of it. God has a time and purpose for each one. If the hour has not yet come, as the pastor concluded, it is almost as if the person can "shake off death." This woman knew she still had something to accomplish, so death could not yet take her. The church is to get behind and support those who for understandable reasons cannot yet say, "It is finished."

Yet sometimes, for reasons we cannot explain, the hour comes when someone has what seems to be an unaccomplished purpose. We asked this pastor about the case of Richard. "Faith and trust are needed because the ultimate decision is reserved in the mind of God. I can't explain why Richard died though he desperately wanted to raise his kids. Neither can I explain why this woman is on her bed nine times, with the doctors saying she is going to die, but she doesn't."

As we shepherd souls through serious illness, Christians should ask the ill person if they have any sense of unfulfilled purpose. It is a discernment question to guide between seeking life and letting go. Yet even when there is a strong sense of unfulfilled purpose, spiritual care reminds the sick that only God fully knows our purpose on earth and that our ultimate purpose is to be with God. All else needs to be entrusted to a loving God whose purpose will be completed.

In addition to contemplating life purpose, there are other questions of spiritual discernment that often help the seriously ill know if it is time to say, "It is finished."

- Are you feeling at peace with God? Do you feel ready to meet him when the time comes?
- Is there anyone you feel led to forgive, or someone you'd like to make peace with?
- Are there any fears or worries on your heart that you'd like to share or talk through?
- Is there anything unfinished, something important to you, that you feel called to complete before death?

When Lois received news that her cancer was incurable, she diligently pursued cancer therapies to extend her life. Despite these efforts, her cancer treatments became increasingly burdensome and the things she loved most—such as dance and her friendships—were lost or diminishing. She knew about hospice care, but her biggest fear was dying alone. We did not have to ask Lois about this fear; she freely volunteered it. After we extended an invitation for her to live in our house for in-home hospice care, she immediately agreed. Lois was not seeking to extend life; she simply couldn't bear the thought of being alone. After this fear was addressed, she readily chose hospice care. As soon as we engaged a key obstacle, Lois was ready to accept her dying.

There is a difficult discernment between seeking life and accepting death. Our death-denying culture makes this especially hard. Christian spiritual care is most effective through an awareness of the obstacles and inner struggles often at work. Those of us who accompany the dying must shepherd gently, tenderly raising spiritual questions and, where the Spirit provides clear openings, offering small nudges toward acceptance and letting go. We walk alongside people with patience and prayer, trusting that the Spirit will move hearts. Letting go is always a personal decision, but the church is called to nurture a faith that, when the time comes, can with Christ say, "It is finished."

Richard's Last Amen

When Patrick arrived in Richard's hospital room, Richard was angrily speaking to the hospitalist physician. She had told him he was not a candidate for the phase 1 clinical trial he was hoping to do as a result of his poor clinical condition, and he was irate.

Patrick interrupted Richard and commanded, "Richard, stop. Now."

Richard looked at Patrick, stunned, and was quiet.

Patrick spoke again, "Everyone, please give Richard and me the room. I need a few moments to privately talk to my friend."

The hospitalist nodded and left the room, followed by his wife, Richard's nurse, and the medical assistant. Patrick sat on the chair next to Richard's bed.

Leaning forward and looking Richard in the eye, he spoke plainly, one former hockey player to another. "What the [ ] are you doing?" he said sternly. "These people are trying to help you. This is not who you are."

It was the kind of talk shaped by their locker-room experiences: tough, direct, and unsentimental. It was intense but not angry or unloving.

Richard paused. And then the truth spilled out: "I'm scared. My body isn't cooperating. Nothing is." His voice trembled. "And my family . . ."

"You have to entrust them to God," Patrick said softly. "God loves them even more than you do. And you need to let these people help you." Then after a pause he continued, "Richard, I want you to hear me clearly: I think his time for you has come."

Richard began to respond but then fell silent as the words reverberated in his mind and soul.

When the family and medical team reentered the room an hour later, something had shifted. Richard was no longer defiant. He asked questions, listened, nodded. He agreed, finally, to hospice care at home.

Days later, he emailed Patrick. He thanked him. He admitted that he needed those words, needed to be humbled. "I know I'm not going to get better," he wrote. "And I accept that now."

Twenty-five days after that meeting, Richard died quietly at home, surrounded by his family and children. In his final days, when Patrick called, Richard no longer had strength to speak. His wife held the phone to his ear. Patrick recited the Lord's Prayer one last time with his friend.

On the other end, barely audible, came a single word of faith from Richard. "Amen."

Nine

Forgiveness

Father, forgive them, for they know not what they do.

Luke 23:34

Without forgiveness there really is no future. . . . Forgiving means abandoning your right to pay back the perpetrator in his own coin, but it is a loss that liberates the victim.

Desmond Tutu

The Seed Beneath

Lois was painstakingly meticulous. Living with her was like hosting a neurotic dinner guest who never left. From the moment she moved in, we began to understand just how particular life would become. It was not always easy.

The tea had to be Earl Grey and only from Trader Joe's. Sweetened exclusively with stevia. Never sugar or Sweet'N Low. No honey. Just stevia.

"And not just any stevia," she reminded us, squinting from behind her ever-present tennis visor, "the one in the green box, with the 'natural' label."

That first morning, we tore through our cabinets looking for it. Nothing. Perhaps muttering a bit, we said, "We'll make a special trip." And we did. Then another. Eventually, we stocked up on all the specialty items. After Lois passed, we gave it all away, stevia included.

Her favorite meal was a fried hot dog with Boston baked beans. It smelled good, but it was definitely not part of our typical diet.

"It reminds me of my father," she'd once admitted. "We used to eat it together every Saturday for dinner. It was our shared ritual."

But it wasn't just about food. Underneath the routines and the color-coded notebooks tied with rubber bands was something deeper. Her habits weren't just preferences. They were protections. Fear, dressed up as control. She didn't just like structure; she depended on it. Every visit, appointment, or phone call Lois meticulously logged, confirmed, and rechecked. Her days were built from these rituals, as if the order itself could keep her from unraveling. And for a while, it did. But at night, something in her softened.

Tracy was usually the one who walked her to the bathroom—fifteen steps, one at a time. She'd also make sure that all the medicine prescribed by hospice had been taken. Lois loved having Tracy as her in-home physician. For every question, every ache, Lois could receive medically informed answers in an unrushed setting. We were careful to never have Tracy prescribe medications, though being trained in both oncology and palliative care made her quick to recognize Lois's medical needs.

Then came the nightly sequence with me (Michael).

I'd fluff the pillows, turn her body just right with pillows pushed under her back, pull up the blanket, tilt the bed, and finally, hold her hand for prayer. This routine took longer than we preferred, so typically Tracy would go to bed, and I would close out the night.

"Will you pray for me?" she'd whisper with her big smile.

"Yes, of course."

"Would you mind saying it out loud?"

So, kneeling beside the bed, Michael and Lois began their routine of nightly prayers.

"God, please grant Lois peace tonight. Let her know she is safe. That you are near."

Almost every night she would interrupt the prayer, first with her fingers tightening around my hands. "Do you really think God could accept someone like me?"

Sometimes the questions came slowly, cautiously. Other nights, they spilled out all at once.

"I want to go to heaven. But I'm not sure if I will."

"Why not?" I asked.

"I've lived for control. Not for him. What if I missed my chance?"

"No one is beyond his reach," I would remind her. "The Lord is gracious. That's the whole point."

On another night, while we were both with her, she surprised us.

"Do you know that song by Bette Midler? 'The Rose'?"

Tracy smiled. "Yeah. My mom used to play it when I was little."

Lois started humming. Then, in a thin, trembling voice, she softly sang the first few words.

She paused, eyes full of tears. "That line . . . about the soul afraid of dying that never learns to live. I think that's me."

Once again Lois caught us by surprise. So much for going to bed anytime soon.

Tracy responded, "Can you tell us more?"

Then Lois reflected, "I danced on stage professionally. But I've never danced with God. I've always felt too unforgiveable."

There was a long silence. Standing on either side of the bed, we each held her hands.

And then I said, "It's not too late, Lois."

Foundations of Forgiveness

The movement from unforgiveness to forgiveness is rooted in Christ. Jesus does not merely model forgiveness; he enacts, initiates, and secures it on behalf of all who trust in him. When he says from the cross, "Father, forgive them," he is not only offering mercy to his executioners but inaugurating a new era of human-divine and human-human reconciliation.

Forgiveness costs something. Spiritually, every sin is a debt against God. "Against you, you only, have I sinned and done what is evil in your sight" (Ps. 51:4), the psalmist confesses. Whether through actions, words, or withheld love, sin violates the character of God and mars God's image among those he has made. Yet, instead of demanding repayment from the sinner, God offers to pay the debt himself. At the cross, Christ bears the full weight of divine justice so that mercy may be freely given.

Uplifting the expansiveness and sufficiency of God's mercy is vital when walking with someone nearing death. Many, consciously or unconsciously, hold that God's favor must be earned. As death approaches, failings throughout life come into greater focus even as the inability to undo or repay them becomes an unavoidable reality. This clash with reality—a reality always present but often obscured by a gossamer veil of lifeless idols woven by the lie of this life's permanence—is terrifying. In the words of T. S. Eliot, "Human kind cannot bear very much reality."[1] The overwhelming darkness of sin can be penetrated only by the light of God's flooding grace in the blood of Christ. "Truly, truly, I say to you, unless you eat the flesh of the Son of Man and drink his blood, you have no life in you" (John 6:53). As we accompany those who are dying, our aim is to grow assurance in the abounding grace of God and the sufficiency of Christ's blood. Jesus said, "It is finished." Our role is to help the dying rest by faith in the glorious completeness of Jesus's work.

Forgiveness is rooted in the character of God as Father. Many carry distorted images of God from earthly experiences, such as distant parents, conditional love, or perfectionist parenting. The distant father figure was the image with which Lois struggled. Though important at any life stage, identifying distorted conceptions of God and uplifting the true God who loves and forgives perfectly is critical to the journey with serious illness.

Over the past twenty-five years, research in geriatric medicine, oncology, and palliative care highlights just how essential forgiveness is in helping individuals cope, heal, and find peace.

In a national survey of 339 palliative care nurses, 87 percent reported that patients or family members expressed deep regret or a desire for forgiveness near the end of life.[2] Similarly, in a large-scale study of advanced cancer patients, over 90 percent identified "forgiveness for sins" as one of their most urgent spiritual needs.[3]

Though primarily spiritual, the experience of forgiveness is linked to emotional and physical well-being. For example, forgiveness has been consistently linked to better mental health. In a longitudinal study of more than fifty thousand adults, those who reported higher levels of forgiveness experienced lower levels of depression, anxiety, and loneliness, and greater emotional well-being.[4] Among cancer survivors, higher forgiveness scores correlated with reduced psychological distress and improved quality of life.[5] Physically, forgiveness supports healing in part through stress reduction. Among individuals living with HIV, higher forgiveness levels were associated with better self-rated health—an association fully mediated by lower stress levels.[6] In people living with heart disease, therapy centered on forgiveness reduced the harmful effects of stress on the heart. In another study, patients with chronic pain who held on to resentment reported higher pain intensity and lower quality of life.[7]

One of the leading international scholars on forgiveness is Christian psychologist Everett Worthington.[8] He conceptualizes forgiveness across three dimensions: with God, with oneself, and with others. In the context of serious illness, attending to forgiveness in one or more of these dimensions is essential for the seriously ill and for those caring for them.

Dimension 1: Forgiveness from God

The sick, and the spiritual caregivers serving them, should prayerfully consider needs for forgiveness from God. For example, many experience feelings of abandonment, punishment, or anger in relation to God. Such burdensome emotions, often left unspoken and unnamed, can be shifted through a spiritual intervention of forgiveness. When these feelings are more specifically explored and named, underlying distortions of God can emerge and be addressed. Consider these statements and the distorted conceptions of God they reveal:

- "Maybe this illness is what I deserve. I've made too many mistakes for God to ignore." (God is a harsh, unforgiving judge.)
- "I don't think God pays attention to people like me anymore; it's like he wound things up and walked away." (God is a distant, unloving Creator.)
- "If this is part of God's plan, I wish I knew why he needs to make it hurt so much." (God is an angry Father.)
- "Other people pray and get healed . . . I guess I'm just not one of his chosen ones." (God is an unloving, unjust parent.)
- "Maybe God's trying to teach me something, but I wish he'd just tell me what it is instead of dragging it out like this." (God is an unloving teacher.)

While each conversation is unique, we must pray for and rely on the Spirit to remove distortions and to illuminate the true nature of God's character afresh, especially to highlight his forgiveness of our sins accomplished through the cross.

Peter was dying in the hospital, but he could not accept that his life was coming to an end. He wanted to live. Only a few weeks earlier, he had still been playing tennis and billiards with his friends every day at the country club. He taped his urinary drainage bag to his inner thigh and wore loose clothing so no one would notice. After each win, he would shake his opponent's hand and then, with a feigned Russian accent, say, "Strong like bull." It was never clear whether he meant himself or the person he had just beaten.

Toward the end, his determination to keep playing sometimes caused the bag to leak onto his shorts and socks. His friends were less bothered by the interruption than they were impressed by his refusal to give in to bladder cancer. Peter had been the senior club champion at tennis for several years and, now in his early seventies, he intended to defend his title again.

That same refusal to let go also kept him from addressing an urgent need to reconcile with a family member. His denial allowed him to stay busy and focus on small goals and daily routines, but it kept him from seeing that death was approaching.

Then his health declined abruptly, and he was admitted to the hospital again. It was his fourth hospitalization that year. He had no intention of it being his last, but it was.

A few days before his death, I (Michael) visited him in his hospital room. I had seen him during a previous hospitalization months earlier. That visit had felt hopeful. He had been alert and energized when I arrived. This time was different. In all the years I had known Peter, I had never seen "the bull" so weak. I wondered if he was near the end.

"How can I pray for you?" I asked.

"Pray that my faith is strengthened," Peter whispered. "I do not know if God will accept me."

His words surprised me. We had talked about faith many times. Peter had become a Christian in his fifties. After that, he became involved in church and Bible study, and he quit drinking.

I felt prompted to ask a simple question I had learned years earlier, one often used when time is short. "Peter, if you were standing before God and he asked you, 'Why should I let you into heaven?' what would you say?"

"That is exactly my fear," Peter said. "I do not think God will let me in. I do not deserve it."

I wondered to myself if Peter's unresolved relationship with his adult son was feeding his guilt and doubt. The brokenness of that relationship may have shaped how he understood his standing before God. His difficulty admitting failure or asking his son for forgiveness was not only relational but spiritual. It pointed to a deeper struggle to trust in the fullness of God's grace. The same reluctance that kept him from confession with his son may have carried into his prayer life, leaving him unsure whether forgiveness could truly reach him. When read through regret rather than mercy, Scripture may have deepened his fear that his failures as a father put him at risk of rejection.

"Peter," I said, "none of us deserve to stand before God. He is the only perfect Father. The rest of us have made many mistakes." I was alluding to his own status as a father without directly saying so. I continued, "The only answer I know is to admit you are not worthy and to ask to enter heaven based on God's grace and the finished work of Jesus on the cross."

"Yes," Peter whispered. "That is what I will say. I trust the blood of Jesus. I believed then, and I believe now. I am just so tired. Please pray that my faith will be strengthened."

I held his hand and prayed with him. Then I said goodbye. When I stepped into the hallway, I could not hold back my tears. I believe I will see Peter again. Still, it is overwhelming to be in a situation when grace, forgiveness, and death are all intertwined.

The beauty of grace flowing through the tragedy of sin and death touches the core of our humanity.

Dimension 2: Forgiving Oneself

Forgiving oneself begins with receiving God's forgiveness while also taking responsibility for the wrongs one has done. It involves treating oneself with compassion rather than continued punishment. Self-forgiveness is essential for finding peace and being released from the suffering caused by unresolved guilt. Without it, a person can spiral downward in ongoing self-condemnation and shame.

Forgiving oneself is rooted in divine forgiveness. By trusting in the words and actions of Jesus and believing that forgiveness is offered through Christ, a person may begin to accept that past wrongdoing is forgiven by God. If God is willing in Christ to forgive me, how can I not come to know that forgiveness myself, despite what I have done? Yet deep trauma and moral injury can make acceptance difficult. Those who have committed serious harm or violence may especially struggle to believe that Jesus's forgiveness applies to them.

Everett Worthington's approach involves six key steps that guide a person from honest responsibility and repair toward self-acceptance, emotional release, and living with new intention. These steps are available in a free online work that can be worked through individually. Additionally, a spiritual caregiver may quietly draw on these concepts within conversation.[9] In the context of illness or end-of-life care, having someone gently support these steps through a loving presence and thoughtful questions can help a person move toward forgiveness and a deeper sense of peace.

This six-step process is illustrated below through a composite narrative drawn from the literature, portraying a veteran's interaction with a hospital chaplain during his final days. The veteran is dying of alcoholism, visible in his gaunt frame and yellowed skin, and the vignette demonstrates how his end-of-life care may address moral injury, war-related trauma, and spiritual struggle.

When the chaplain had visited Bob the day before, their conversation had been light. They spoke briefly about faith, then spoke mostly about sports, laughing together about another winning streak by the New England Patriots.

When the chaplain returned the next morning, the veteran's mood had altered. He nodded in greeting but did not turn his head. His eyes remained fixed out the window. After a long silence, he spoke in a raspy whisper.

"I can see their faces. The ones I killed in Vietnam."

The chaplain leaned forward in his chair and stayed silent.

"I see them when I close my eyes," Bob said softly. "They were just kids. I don't know how to die like this . . . with that on me."

Before forgiveness can begin, there must be a place to bring the truth. The chaplain had noticed the check mark by "Catholic" in Bob's chart. He also had a cross tattooed on his right forearm. The first step is receiving forgiveness from the Sacred. It is not about excusing but about opening the heart to God's mercy.

"You're not beyond grace," the chaplain said gently. "Have you spoken to Christ, who knows you fully and still offers mercy?"

Bob hesitated, then closed his eyes. His left hand grasped his right forearm.

The chaplain did not ask, but he wondered what memories lived in that arm.

"God . . . I'm sorry," Bob whispered, his left hand now squeezing his right forearm.

His body shook with grief. After a long silence, his hands dropped to his sides and he drew a deep, uneven breath. It was likely the first breath in a long time that was not gripped by shame.

"You've taken the first step," the chaplain said quietly. "Not to erase the past, but to stop letting it destroy who you are."

Bob, now visibly crying, said, "I wish I could tell them. Say I'm sorry."

Repairing relationships is the second step in forgiveness. Sometimes this happens through direct words or actions. Other times, especially at the end of life, repair can only take symbolic or inward forms. What matters is the desire to honor those harmed and to take responsibility where possible.

"Maybe in the next life you'll be given that chance," the chaplain said. "And if so, I imagine there will be joy."

"That's a new thought," the veteran replied, after gathering himself and wiping his tears from his eyes. "I thought I'd never have a chance to make it right."

"You can still honor them now," the chaplain said. "You can name them. Light a candle for each face you remember. God knows their names. God knows your remorse." Trying to make amends is the third step.

The fourth step of forgiveness involves quieting the mind when it becomes trapped in self-punishment. This does not mean suppressing memories but learning to hold them without being crushed by them. The veteran did not yet speak of this directly, but the softening of his body and his steadier breathing suggested that the grip of rumination had slightly eased.

The chaplain continued, "I'm not making excuses, but you were a young man in the fog of war. You can grieve and still allow yourself to be forgiven."

The veteran turned his eyes toward the chaplain, holding his gaze for the first time.

"I don't want to be remembered for what I did," he said. "Just that I tried to make it right before it was too late."

Accepting oneself as flawed but still worthy is the fifth step in self-forgiveness. It allows a person to release the need for punishment and to die with dignity rather than condemnation.

"Sometimes it helps to speak to your younger self," the chaplain said. "To tell him what you know now, with honesty and compassion." This kind of practice, often called imaginal dialogue, allows forgiveness to move from an idea into an embodied emotional experience.

"I'm willing to try," Bob said. "But not today. I think I need some time to rest."

The final step of forgiving self is living with intention in whatever time remains. It does not require grand actions. Sometimes it is simply choosing truth and peace.

The following day when the chaplain returned, Bob eagerly shared some ways he had been working on the things they had discussed. Something had shifted. It was clear that Bob's vise-grip of guilt had finally loosened.

Dimension 3: Forgiving Others

Interpersonal forgiveness is an inward turning away from ill will toward someone who has caused harm and a movement toward goodwill.[10] It is different from reconciliation, which requires truth telling, repentance, and meaningful repair between people. Forgiveness does not excuse abuse or deny sin. Instead, it frees the wounded person from resentment and the desire for revenge, entrusting justice to God.

Reconciliation depends on the offender's repentance, but forgiveness can be offered even when the other person is unwilling, unavailable, or has passed away. A person may forgive before God without restoring the relationship. This kind of forgiveness releases the heart from bitterness and opens space for peace. Jesus speaks plainly about the cost of refusing forgiveness, warning, "If you do not forgive others their trespasses, neither will your Father forgive your trespasses" (Matt. 6:15). This is not a threat, but a loving warning that unforgiveness binds the soul.

Forgiveness is a common theme at life's end, with more than half of patients contemplating forgiveness[11] and unresolved hurt.[12] Many desire reconciliation before death. In one hospice study, nearly half the patients died peacefully within forty-eight hours of resolving key relationships.[13]

Throughout life and especially near life's end, forgiveness can bring relief, peace, and even restoration. We should prayerfully pursue forgiveness of others, ideally with trusted spiritual supporters and always with God's help. Approaches such as Worthington's REACH model provide practical steps that facilitate movement from decisional to emotional forgiveness.[14]

The REACH Model of Forgiveness

R	Recall the hurt	Acknowledge the wrong committed and the related pain, without dwelling on it.
E	Empathize	Seek to understand the circumstances and emotions that shaped the action, cultivating compassion without excusing the harm.
A	Altruistic gift of forgiveness	Choose to forgive as a gift, offering mercy rather than waiting for forgiveness to be earned.
C	Commit to forgiveness	Make a clear and intentional decision to forgive, expressed privately or through a simple act such as prayer or writing.
H	Hold on to forgiveness	Return to the decision when guilt or shame returns, remembering that forgiveness is a practice over time.

Table is adapted from Everett L. Worthington, *Forgiving and Reconciling: Bridges to Wholeness and Hope* (InterVarsity, 2003), 73.

Based on Worthington's REACH model, the Human Flourishing Program at Harvard University adapted interpersonal forgiveness exercises into a workbook for use in churches.[15] Working through these exercises personally is an important step before helping others forgive.

Some gentle ways to begin, whether for self-reflection or in spiritual care of others, is to ask questions such as

"Have you been thinking about forgiveness, for yourself or for others?"

"Is there anyone you'd like to make peace with?"

"Is there something you'd like to let go of before you leave this earth?"

When a sick person holds unforgiveness toward someone who has harmed them, spiritual care helps them consider how this burden affects their soul. Being sinned against can leave a person holding anger, bitterness, and resentment. Forgiveness is not denial of harm but a way of releasing oneself from its grip. It is an action modeled after Christ (Luke 23:34), who calls us to forgive others (Matt. 18:35; Luke 6:37). Through prayer and gentle guidance, the person is invited to name the injury honestly, acknowledge the pain it caused, and choose to release the offender into God's care. Forgiveness becomes a decision made before God in prayer, and it is often an ongoing emotional process. While the past cannot be changed, and God holds all unrepentant sin accountable, forgiveness allows the wounded person to move from being trapped by harm to becoming free, restored, and able to live or die with greater peace.

Others are in need of forgiveness for harms they have committed, such as Bob, who was haunted by harms he committed during the Vietnam War. If the person (or persons) harmed is still living, the sick person should consider some expression of sincere apology, such as writing a letter or making a phone call. Here the counsel of a pastor or other spiritual supporter can help guide how to ask for forgiveness in a manner sensitive to the relationship and the needs of the person harmed. Sometimes there is no way to directly seek the forgiveness of those harmed, such as was the case for Bob. Here as well, the counsel of a trusted spiritual caregiver can be critical to consider how to express remorse and seek forgiveness in other ways, even if only to do so before God.

Forgiveness and reconciliation, as related but distinct concepts, cannot be forced. They require movement of the Spirit to bring forth honesty and humility from the one who caused harm and courage to let go of injustice from the one who was hurt. By the Spirit's enabling, we are called to share in, and to receive, Jesus's prayer, "Father, forgive them, for they know not what they do."

A Return Home

The day before Peter's death, his middle-aged son, Kevin, got a call from a family member about his dad's imminent decline. Kevin flew across the country, knowing it might be the end. A few years earlier, Kevin confronted his father about the pain and abandonment he felt following his parents' divorce. But Peter had rebuffed Kevin's words, retorting that he was desperately escaping a difficult and painful marriage and was just trying to survive emotionally. He wasn't ready to admit fault or ask for forgiveness. That conversation left Kevin feeling more hurt than before.

Despite their painful disagreement, they maintained more contact than beforehand. And despite Kevin's lingering sense of abandonment, he still wanted to see his father and say goodbye.

When Kevin walked into the hospital room, he saw the emaciated face of the man who, in all his memories, had been strong and athletic. Peter's eyes filled with tears, and the two held hands. Peter couldn't speak, but his eyes said everything. Aware that there was still unresolved tension, one of the family members gently asked the rest of the family to step out and give father and son a few moments alone.

"Dad, I want you to know that I love you very much," Kevin began. "You've been a good dad. I've especially loved our conversations over the past few years. We made up for some lost time."

Peter could only hold Kevin's hand and look into his eyes. His grip tightened, and Kevin could still feel the old bull's strength.

"Before everyone comes back," Kevin continued, "I need to say something. Even if you don't think it's necessary, I want you to know that I forgive you. I understand more clearly now how hard your marriage to Mom was. While we can't get those years back, I've let it all go. I'm just grateful to have this last chance to say I love you."

With tears streaming down his face, Peter silently mouthed, "I love you," then gathered his strength and spoke clearly, "my son."

Though Peter never admitted fault or asked for forgiveness, Kevin's words seemed to bring healing to them both. Love covers over and brings healing to our wounds (1 Pet. 4:8).

Those facing serious illness, and those who are privileged to be with the seriously ill, should seek and support forgiveness. Gently prompting forgiveness with God, with oneself, and with others lies at the heart of preparing for dying and accompanying the ill on their journey home.

"The Rose"

"I think I was always afraid," Lois whispered. "I knew how to move with a partner on the dance floor . . . but not with God. I didn't think I could trust him not to drop me."

Lois and I (Michael) had been having these kinds of conversations for nearly two months, almost every night. Just before bedtime, the deeper questions surfaced: about her failed marriage, friends who had disappeared, and her unfulfilled hope of selling the video art she created while finishing a master's degree at the Museum of Fine Arts in Boston.

Lois was instinctively conducting her own life review. Again and again, her questions circled back to God.

"Michael, do you really think God could love someone like me?"

"Yes, Lois," I said. "I do. Not because you've earned it. Because that's who he is."

She thought about that. I could see it in her eyes. And then one night, she said it.

"Do you think it would be too strange . . . if I got baptized here? In this bed?"

I looked at her gently. "Not strange," I said. "But Lois, are you sure? Is this something you really want? There's no pressure from me or anyone else."

She let out a big breath, then gave that little half-smile of hers. "Oh Michael. No one could make me do anything I don't want to do. You know that. This is from my heart."

Then her eyes lit up just a little. "You know how we have been playing the song 'The Rose'?"

I nodded.

"I think I've been that seed. Frozen," she said. Then with a beaming smile she looked me in the eyes. "But I think spring is finally coming."

The afternoon of April 15, 2021, was unseasonably warm. A dozen people from church gathered in Lois's room—those who had visited, prayed, and read Scripture with her over the past months. One of her former dance partners stood near the window. Tracy and I had made space around her bed. She wore her tennis visor, and a light scarf around her shoulders. A little blush touched her cheeks. She looked tired, but radiant.

We sang "Amazing Grace," voices filling the bedroom. After the song, I spoke the words of a simple baptismal liturgy. Lois had said she didn't want to speak too much, just enough to make it clear to the Lord that this was her act of faith.

"Lois," I asked, "is it in fact your decision, and your decision alone, to present yourself for Christian baptism today?"

She nodded. "Yes," she said clearly, "this is my heart's desire."

"Have you placed your faith in Christ's death on the cross, trusting him to forgive all your sins—past, present, and future?"

"Yes," she said, "by his grace, I believe in Christ's cross."

"And do you believe in your heart that God raised Jesus from the dead, and that through him you have the hope of eternal life?"

"Yes," she said slowly and with a clear, confident voice, "by his grace, I believe."

I took a small bowl of water and gently poured it over her forehead.

"In the name of the Father, and of the Son, and of the Holy Spirit, Lois Ann Meinhardt, you are baptized into the death and resurrection of Jesus Christ."

She closed her eyes and smiled.

Someone near the foot of the bed whispered, "Thank you, Lord."

Her old dance partner stepped forward after the prayer, leaned down, and kissed her hand.

"You never stopped dancing, Lois. You just changed partners."

That night, after everyone had gone, Tracy and I sat beside her once more. She took our hands. But this time, she didn't ask any questions.

"Why don't you pray and then I'll pray," she suggested.

It was a subtle but wonderful shift. The seed of forgiveness was beginning to bloom, like a rose in spring.

Ten

Medicine, Pain, and Hope

Jesus called out with a loud voice, "Father, into your hands I commit my spirit."

Luke 23:46 NIV

To place the hope of one's health in the hands of the doctor is the act of an irrational animal. This, nevertheless, is what we observe in the case of certain unhappy persons who do not hesitate to call their doctors their "saviors." Yet, to reject entirely the benefits to be derived from this art is the sign of a pettish nature. . . . So, then, we should neither repudiate this art altogether nor does it behoove us to repose all our confidence in it; . . . when reason allows, we call in the doctor, but we do not leave off hoping in God.

St. Basil the Great

All shall be well, and all shall be well, and every kind of thing shall be well.

Julian of Norwich

Bleeding for My Sins

On a humid Saturday evening in Boston, Sharon Watson, a forty-three-year-old woman from Dorchester, arrived at the emergency department with heavy vaginal bleeding. For more than six months she had noticed spotting between her cycles, but the past week had brought on a flood—soaking through three to four pads a day. Alongside the bleeding, she had noticed how easily she became short of breath. Just walking up the single flight of stairs to her apartment made her feel winded. A grocery store clerk by day and caregiver for her two young grandchildren by night, Sharon hadn't had the time or resources to see a doctor.

At the hospital, blood tests showed she was anemic consistent with her bleeding. On her physical exam, the gynecological resident discovered a large cervical mass, and further imaging confirmed advanced-stage cervical cancer. Sharon received two units of blood and was admitted for further care. When Dr. Kearney, the attending gynecologic oncologist, came to her hospital room to discuss treatment, Sharon was surrounded by her daughter and several church friends. A Bible lay open on her side table; spiritual get-well cards lined her windowsill.

Dr. Kearney, standing at Sharon's bedside, folded her arms across her white coat as she introduced herself. She then began to explain her cancer and its treatment. "Ms. Watson, based on the size of the tumor and where it's spread, this is stage IIIB cervical cancer. With treatment—if it's done on time and without interruption—your chance for cure is about 30 percent. That might sound low, but it's real. The key is starting right away and coming for your treatments without interruption. You'll have daily radiation for about seven weeks, and chemotherapy happens once a week during your radiation therapy. Some of your radiation will be delivered by a surgical procedure called brachytherapy. We'll be getting you started here in the hospital, but you'll be able to receive treatments from home after a week or so. This is tough treatment, but we will support you through it and give you the best chance of cure possible. Remember, delays in your treatment lower your chances for cure considerably."

Sharon held her gaze, then gently interrupted. "Doctor, I have a question. Do you hear from God?"

Caught off guard, Dr. Kearney hesitated. "I'm sorry, I don't think I understand your question. I don't hear God as far as I know."

"God's talking to you all the time," Sharon replied with confidence.

Not knowing how best to respond, Dr. Kearney paused and shifted on her feet while unfolding her arms and placing her hands in her white coat pockets. She then replied, "Ms. Watson, I'm your doctor, not a priest."

Sharon's eyes held steady. "You might not hear him, but he is always talking to all of us. All you have to do is listen."

After a long pause, Dr. Kearney nodded her head and said, "Okay." She then redirected the conversation back to her treatment, asking, "Do you have any questions about the radiation and chemotherapy? I'm hoping to get you started in the next day or two."

Sharon nodded slowly. "I'm going to pray on it. Jesus is the one driving. My hope is in him. I'm just in the back seat going for the ride."

Though she started treatment in the hospital, Sharon began missing radiation appointments once discharged. Some days she came late; others, not at all. When Dr. Kearney pressed her about the importance of staying on schedule, Sharon responded with a question of her own.

"Doctor, are you a believing person?"

Dr. Kearney looked up from her computer. "I wouldn't say I'm religious."

"That's not what I'm asking," Sharon replied. "I'm asking, do you know Jesus?"

The doctor gave a nervous laugh. "I grew up Catholic, but that doesn't matter. I'm your doctor, and my job is to treat your cancer. That's why I'm encouraging you to come to every one of your treatments—so we can most effectively treat your cancer."

Sharon nodded and after a pause said, "I'll do my best to be here."

One Sunday after service, in the middle of Sharon's seven-week treatment, Sister Gloria, a longtime church elder and beloved member of Sharon's congregation, found Sharon sitting quietly at the back of the fellowship hall. Sharon hadn't stayed for lunch or prayer, but Sister Gloria felt led to sit beside her.

"Child, I heard you've been missing some of your treatments," Sister Gloria said gently, placing a hand on Sharon's shoulder.

Sharon gave a slow nod. "It's hard, Sister Gloria. The fatigue. Watching the babies. Sometimes I just feel like maybe this is all just . . ." Her eyes began to water. "Maybe God is punishing me for the things I did in the old days, before I got saved."

Sister Gloria took her hand warmly. "Oh honey, don't let the enemy put that lie in your head. This isn't punishment—it's just life. And life brings trials. But you've already been washed clean by his blood. Don't forget that."

Tears filled Sharon's eyes. "As soon as I saw the bleeding, I said to myself that I was bleeding for my sins."

Sister Gloria looked her in the eyes, steady and calm. "His blood paid it all. You have to have positivity and stay away from the negativity. You got to stay away from the shoulda, coulda, woulda. Okay? Our hope is built on nothing less than Christ's righteousness. That's how you keep walking forward in hope. Not by what you did, but by what he's doing in you now."

Sharon exhaled deeply, her shoulders loosening just a bit.

"We're going to help you through this," Sister Gloria continued. "Your church family is here. We'll get you rides. Watch the babies if we have to. But you've got to show up for your healing. You hear me?"

After that conversation, Sharon came for every appointment without fail. For her final week of radiation, Sharon was hospitalized. The pain was severe, but she refused more than minimal pain medication. Concerned, her night nurse asked the hospital chaplain to visit.

The next day, Chaplain Betsy found Sharon alone, gazing out the window. Sharon agreed to talk.

"How are you holding up?" Betsy asked gently.

"I'm all right," Sharon answered, her voice thin. "Just tired. The pain comes in waves."

"I heard you've been avoiding pain medication. May I ask why?"

Sharon looked at her sharply, then softened. "Because I'm not going back. I used to be hooked on everything—pills, crack, whatever I could get. It nearly ruined me. Took everything from me—my babies, my mind, my soul. I worked too hard, prayed too hard to be clean. I'd rather feel every bit of this pain than go back to that darkness."

Betsy nodded solemnly. "That takes incredible strength."

"It's not me," Sharon said. "It's Jesus. He pulled me out of that mess. I was that woman at his feet, crying my soul out. And he picked me up. I owe him everything. So no, no pain pills. I can handle this pain. What I can't handle is being chained again."

They sat together in silence for a moment.

Sharon continued, her voice stronger. "When the bleeding started, I knew something was wrong. But I also knew God was preparing me. On June 4, Sister Gloria laid hands on me during that Sunday celebration, and I felt the Spirit like fire in my bones. Six days later, I got my diagnosis. That wasn't a coincidence. That was God telling me, 'I've got you.'"

Sharon squeezed her eyes shut as a wave of pain surged. Then the tension eased and she could breathe again. "My life is in his hands. If I take that medicine, it means I've given in. But he's not letting go of me, and I ain't letting go of him."

Hope Has the Last Word

After the separation Jesus expressed during the moment of cosmic darkness, "My God, my God, why have you forsaken me?" (Mark 15:34), the final words of Jesus at his death are accented by hope: "Then Jesus, calling out with a loud voice, said, 'Father, into your hands I commit my spirit!' And having said this he breathed his last" (Luke 23:46). These final words powerfully convey reconnection and restoration of hope. Rather than "my God," Jesus readdresses him as "Father," pointing to their restored relationship. Even though his body is dying, Jesus fully trusts that his spirit will be received by the hands of the Father. Death is not the end. The last words of Jesus ring with hope for a good future that is held in the capable hands of the Father.

These words are a model and a lesson for those who are sick and their caregivers to hold on to hope. No matter what is happening with your body, it is not the end. This hope for a good future that is held in God's all-powerful hands drives out all fear and hopelessness.

Reclaiming God's Gift of Medicine

One of the more significant disjunctions between contemporary medicine and the church arises from a distinct set of hopes. While Christians emphasize the centrality of hoping in God, there can be a subtle or sometimes overt emphasis in secular medicine to put hope in medicine's powers to heal. More than a few believers have encountered a spirit of arrogance or self-sufficiency within the medical profession. At times, pastors and faith perspectives are dismissed as antiquated or irrelevant by medical professionals. Not uncommonly, one may encounter a physician whose demeanor suggests a godlike confidence in their own healing powers. This troubling posture is sometimes echoed in institutional rhetoric and hospital slogans that proclaim, for example, "Miracles happen here," or "Depend on us for life."[1] In one advertisement, a patient shares, "It made all the difference to hand myself over to the team with total and unconditional trust." Such messages blur the line between advertisement and religious-sounding faith. For Christians, God alone is the source of miracles, and it is on him that we should ultimately depend. It is false hope to place total and unconditional trust in physicians, medicine, or hospitals. These messages can subtly reinforce a vision of medicine that elevates human powers to the level of God.

Excessive professional pride is not only spiritually unhealthy for the clinician, but it can also fracture the therapeutic alliance between doctor and patient. From a theological standpoint, it is deeply worrisome when Christian patients sense the clinician's posture of self-sufficiency that leaves little room for divine grace. Such encounters can deepen mistrust, particularly for believers seeking holistic care that honors body and soul together.

A case in point is the interaction between Sharon and her physician, Dr. Kearney. Sharon grounds her ultimate hope in God while Dr. Kearney centers on the earthly hopes achievable by medical means. Hence, while Dr. Kearney confidently delivered technical medical information, she failed to truly listen to what Sharon was communicating at a heart level. Sharon was seeking more than clinical information; she was searching for trust, compassion, and a sense of personal connection.

Lois had a similar experience with her medical team at the hospital. She was incessantly questioning her medical caregivers to understand her medical care. In response, the medical staff labeled Lois a "difficult patient." We could see their point, but we also understood that Lois felt alone, vulnerable, and anxious. These emotions fueled her constant questions, which were the outflow of her desire to gain a sense of control over her out-of-control health circumstances. Lois conveyed to us how she could feel her medical team's irritation toward her, which only deepened the disconnection with her medical caregivers and made her feel dehumanized.

Similarly, Dr. Kearney's unwillingness to engage, even modestly, with the spiritual dimension of "Ms. Watson" left Sharon feeling unseen as a person. Ironically, Dr. Kearney's ambivalence toward Sharon's faith led to Sharon feeling less connected and committed to Dr. Kearney's medical plan. Dr. Kearney assumed that Sharon's spiritual questions were irrelevant to her medical care, when in fact they aimed to clarify if Dr. Kearney's medical care was collaborative with, or in competition with, Sharon's understanding of God. Given Sharon's faith in God had already quite literally saved her from a life-threatening disease—drug addiction—her question is understandable. But Dr. Kearney did not recognize this underlying dynamic. Though Dr. Kearney may not have been able to endorse personally hearing from God, she could still signal her respect for, and collaboration with, Sharon's deeply held beliefs by responding with words such as, "I hear that your faith is very important to you. Can you tell me about that?" But instead of forging connection, Dr. Kearney's response inadvertently pitted hope in God against hope in medicine.

It is not the church's role to directly rebuke clinicians who become arrogant or show undue hope in medicine's powers. Rather, faith communities are called to bear witness to a foundational theological truth: All healing, whether through prayer alone or through medical intervention, ultimately comes from God. As Scripture reminds us: "I am the Lord who heals you" (Exod. 15:26 NIV). Sharon was simply following through with what St. Basil had advised centuries before: Christians "call in the doctor, but we do not leave off hoping in God."[2]

A foundational principle undergirding a theological understanding of medicine is that it is a gift from God that often mediates his healing powers.[3] When clinicians recognize and respect this value or themselves affirm this core belief, the therapeutic alliance with their believing patients is strengthened.[4] A patient-clinician relationship rooted in honored spiritual values, whether or not explicitly shared, can remove unnecessary obstacles to holistic care. Conversely, when the patient's core spiritual values are ignored or implicitly denied, the practice of medicine can subtly elevate itself to divine-like status. In such cases, human pride in medicine's powers can become an obstacle in the path of healing for some patients.

Christian clinicians bear a particular opportunity in this regard. By consciously and humbly giving credit to God as the source of healing, they model a right ordering of medical practice within the broader story of divine providence. Sixteenth-century French surgeon Ambroise Paré is quoted as saying to his patients, "I dress wounds, but God heals them."[5] Multiple organizations importantly guide and support trainees and clinicians in how to ethically and professionally integrate faith and practice.[6] In contrast, whenever medical practices are framed independently of the Creator, Christians should recognize this as possible idolatry, a distortion of both theology and medicine. Christian clinicians have a role to play by reminding the church that medicine is temporal and limited. It cannot bring salvation, nor can it hold back death for long. When medicine is effective, true credit goes to the source of healing.

From nearly the beginning of the Christian tradition, followers of Jesus have affirmed the goodness of medicine. The parable of the good Samaritan found in the Gospel of Luke—who himself was a physician (Col. 4:14)—illustrates a compassionate use of medicinal resources, such as oil and wine (Luke 10:34), in the care of the wounded. Jesus himself was known as the Great Physician (see Luke 5:31), a title that honors both the Divine Healer and, by extension, the healing arts.

In the early centuries of the church, leaders like Basil the Great articulated a nuanced understanding of medicine. He warned against placing ultimate hope in bodily health, cautioning the faithful not to fall into a "craze for bodily health." Yet Basil, who himself was trained as a Hippocratic physician, did not reject medicine; rather, he recognized it as a good gift from God—a mercy of God to alleviate some of the consequences of humanity's fall (Gen. 3). God's mercy enables humans to farm despite thorns, to make clothing to cover their nakedness, and to discover medicine for pain. Thus, medicine, rightly received, is an instrument for the alleviation of sickness and the promotion of healing.

Even when clinicians exhibit a spirit of arrogance or express false hope, rather than reacting to that distortion, the church must continue to encourage its people to receive the gift of medicine with discernment and gratitude. It is a tool, not a god. Furthermore, given our myopic tendency to view temporal forms of healing as ultimate goods, the church must continually remind its people that healing in this life is only a foreshadowing of the ultimate healing we will experience in the resurrection. Accordingly, hope is secure through Jesus whether or not bodily healing occurs in this life. Bodily healing, no matter how dramatic or miraculous, is but a raindrop in comparison to the power and vastness of the glorious ocean that is bodily resurrection healing. Temporary bodily healing may come through medicine, but Jesus, the Great Physician, is our true hope for everlasting healing.

Hope Through Pain

Another topic that often arises in spiritual care is how to approach pain and its treatment during illness and near death. For example, some are understandably concerned about overreliance on pain medications, whereas others are anxious and frightened of the possible experience of pain.

In the 1960s, Dame Cicely Saunders, a Christian nurse and physician who founded the hospice movement, set forth the idea of "total pain," which conceptualizes pain as an experience involving the physical, emotional, social, and spiritual dimensions of a person.[7] How each dimension is impacted varies according to circumstances and personalities, but they are each impacted nonetheless. Accordingly, one's faith is intertwined with a pain experience and often serves as a way of coping with pain. For example, in one study of cancer patients, 71 percent agreed with the statement, "My faith helps me to endure the suffering that comes with difficult medical treatments."[8]

According to this multidimensional understanding, embedded within the experience of pain are complex social, emotional, and spiritual interpretations. For example, due to the larger societal awareness of the dangers of pain medications (e.g., addiction, overdose), patients and family members often cite addiction concerns as a reason to avoid use of opioids to control pain within serious illness. This perspective has also been seen among religious leaders who tend to overestimate addiction risks associated with pain medications and to underestimate the effectiveness of managing side effects.[9] Another common social interpretation of pain is that the use of narcotic medications such as morphine means that death is imminent. Other interpretations of pain and its treatment can arise from prior life experiences, such as was the case for Sharon. Sharon's prior experience with addiction resulted in an understandable reluctance to take pain medication.

In addition, her endurance of pain without medication was equated in her mind with reliance on God. Her prior reliance on "pills" had only led to her destruction, whereas reliance on God had brought about her healing. Enduring pain without medication was hence equated with relying on God. Such narratives surrounding pain and other symptoms of illness and treatment can form powerful frameworks of meaning that forge resilience in suffering. Sharon's endurance of severe pain was a powerful manifestation of her deep faith. However, such narratives can also contain distortions that can be harmful. For example, what if Sharon's pain were to exceed what she could handle by non-opiate medications and her spiritual coping skills? Sharon would be forced to choose between holding on to her faith or accepting narcotic pain medications, arguably a distorted dichotomization. Here is where others accompanying the sick can assist by shining light on the complex emotional, social, and spiritual narratives that arise in the experience of suffering, allowing for new interpretations, and even spiritual growth, to be discovered.

Sharon's visit by the hospital chaplain, Betsy, highlights how simple questions can shed light on these complex social, emotional, and spiritual narratives that may arise surrounding the experience of pain and suffering. She asked Sharon simply why she wouldn't take the medication. Probing questions that uncover these underlying narratives can be posed in self-reflection and by pastors and other spiritual supporters to ill persons. Examples include:

- What has this illness meant to you personally?
- How has this illness affected how you see yourself?
- How has your understanding of your illness changed over time?
- What worries you about your illness?
- What are you hoping for as you're dealing with this illness?

Such questions achieve two important goals. First, they uncover and signal care for the deeper experience of the person who is suffering. Pain and other forms of suffering are inherently isolating, and questions aiming to connect with that experience help suffering persons feel valued and less alone. Betsy's conversation with Sharon achieved that. Her question signaled her care and allowed Sharon's story to be heard and honored.

Second, probing questions allow for narratives to be interacted with, particularly where there are potential distortions or places where new interpretations might be helpful. For example, Paul, an elderly Christian man suffering through ongoing medical treatments for his end-stage congestive heart failure, had on multiple occasions expressed resistance to hospice care despite it having been recommended by his doctor. A fellow congregant—also a nurse—asked Paul why he was reluctant to consider hospice care, and he expressed concern about being overly medicated to unconsciousness and death. This prompted a conversation about hospice care and a clarification that led to his willingness to transition to hospice, where he received excellent symptom management and remained lucid until a few days before his death.

Similarly, in Sharon's case, Betsy was able to communicate with her nurse and other members of the medical team the reason underlying her resistance to pain medication. This led to the medical team discussing with Sharon pain management strategies using primarily non-opiate pain medications. They also reassured her by sharing their evidence-based protocol for treating patients' pain with opiates in the context of prior addiction, including by minimizing the use of opiate pain medications, utilizing the lowest effective dose for the shortest time, and monitoring closely.

In contrast to Sharon, Lois viewed her pain quite differently. For her, pain threatened her autonomy. Once she chose hospice care and moved into our home, she committed herself to a strict pain-management plan. If she experienced pain, she was quick to request stronger regulation. I (Tracy) spent many hours advocating for her, ensuring the hospice physician adjusted her medications appropriately. Every Sunday night, I filled Lois's weekly morning and evening pill organizer, measuring out a complicated regimen that demanded vigilance. The counting never stopped. Managing prescriptions became its own burden of care. I was not infrequently on the phone with physicians or pharmacists, and on several occasions, I had to send Michael scurrying to multiple pharmacies around the city to secure various medications. When these efforts failed and medications ran low, Lois's anxiety would skyrocket. She feared discomfort so deeply that even the thought of unmanaged pain was unbearable.

The contrast between Sharon and Lois is remarkable. Sharon viewed her endurance of pain as a spiritual victory, reflecting her reliance upon the God who had saved her. Lois experienced physical suffering as a threat to her autonomy and control—strategies that had long been the framework for her survival of a harsh world as a single, impoverished woman. Both Sharon and Lois were in need of new narratives in their interpretations of pain. Sharon could have reinterpreted pain treatment as God's provision, including the experienced clinicians to ensure it was provided in a manner that didn't rekindle addiction. Lois could have grown in understanding that pain and suffering could not take away her identity, because no matter her circumstances she was beloved and uniquely created by God (Ps. 139:14). She could also have grown in trust that God was present with her in her pain and that he had provided, and would continue to provide, the people and medications needed for her to endure.

From a theological perspective, pain is not part of the original creation but a result of sin (Gen. 3). The narrative of redemption points to a future in the resurrection when there will be no more pain (Rev. 21:4). Whereas we have not yet received the restoration of body or soul, Scripture frames the use of medicinal agents for healing or pain relief in a positive way. For those administering medications to people in pain, the treatment is an act of Christlike compassion (Luke 10:33–34) and gives rest to the weary (Matt. 11:28). Both Proverbs (31:6–7) and the apostle Paul (1 Tim. 5:23) counsel the use of wine for medicinal purposes during illness. Pain alleviation is an act of love and serves as a reminder that God offers comfort to those suffering physical pain. It is not the will of God for his people to agonize in physical pain or to callously dismiss those who are suffering.

When medical and pastoral care came together, both Sharon's and Lois's devotion could be honored and their fears gently addressed. The ill can be reassured that receiving relief from pain is not weakness but an expression of God's mercy. Christ has already suffered for us; because of him, we need not carry unnecessary suffering when relief is possible. Yet not all pain will be removed. In those moments, the virtue of patience is required, and the hope that our brief suffering is joined to Christ's own. As Paul writes, "Now I rejoice in my sufferings for your sake, and in my flesh I am filling up what is lacking in Christ's afflictions" (Col. 1:24). Pain and suffering are indeed evils, but not without meaning. Medicine that eases pain may be received as a gift from God. It is a reminder of the hope of resurrection when there will be no more tears and no more pain. Yet this present suffering reminds us of the hope of the cross each of us is called to bear. Both Sharon and Lois were invited through their suffering to hope in God in new ways, both through his hands of comfort and through the meaning he provides.

Punishment and Suffering

An additional temptation in suffering is to interpret it as God's judgment. Sharon's story exemplifies this common response. As soon as Sharon saw her bleeding, she thought God was punishing her, particularly as the source of her bleeding was associated with the sexual behaviors that surrounded her drug addiction. Unresolved guilt can often lead to such interpretations: If I am getting what I deserve, I should patiently accept the punishment. Some will even refuse curative treatment with the rationale that pursuing medical treatments is a form of resisting God's will.

Illness-as-punishment is a common religious response. In our study of cancer patients in Boston, one out of five (22 percent) cancer patients thought they were being punished by God.[10] In a study of 331 patients at six outpatient palliative care centers, 15 percent of patients thought God was punishing them.[11] In more traditional religious cultures, a belief in God's punishment through illness is higher, including 74 percent among those with sickle cell disease in the West Indies.[12] There is also a tendency for believers to make supernatural attributions to their disease because it provides a rationale for the sickness; sometimes a negative explanation is preferred over no explanation at all.[13]

Yet if we learn nothing else from the cross of Christ, it is that the innocent are often scapegoated and mocked as though they deserve their suffering. The cross rebukes retribution theology by revealing that the innocent not only suffer but are also falsely accused of deserving it. Despite his agony, Jesus's final words on the cross are of hope and an unconditional affirmation of sonship with the Father. The cross teaches believers that suffering should never be quickly equated with the guilty receiving their just deserts.

Scripture's discussion of illness and suffering is that there are many reasons for suffering. Yes, we live in a cause-and-effect world, but like the man born blind, suffering can create opportunities for God's extraordinary love and power to be on display. Additionally, suffering often leads to spiritual growth. It can produce virtues including humility (2 Cor. 12:7–10), patience (James 1:2–4), hope (Rom. 5:2–5), and joy (1 Pet. 1:6–9). In addition, Christ's redemptive suffering is embodied and extended in the experience of Christ's disciples (Rom. 8:17–18; 1 Pet. 4:12–13). There is a unique union with Christ in which the believer shares in his sufferings. Lastly, as we see with Job, there is mystery to it all.

However, we often viscerally resist accepting this mystery, particularly as unexplained suffering leaves us feeling helpless to avoid it. Not uncommonly, we resort to simplistic explanations—including viewing illness as God's judgment—at least in part to make our world seem more controllable. Such explanations often reflect limited or distorted theologies that can prove harmful. For example, Kate Bowler writes poignantly from her own illness experience of how easy Christian explanations for her suffering, such as "Everything happens for a reason," were wounding.[14] There is no spiritual formula for pain, and hope cannot be demanded of the sick. Rather, hope is a gift formed through suffering (Rom. 5:3–5). Julian of Norwich's words "All shall be well" were received by her as a revelation from the Spirit while she lay gravely ill during the Black Plague.[15] In suffering, whether that of others or our own, we must prayerfully identify and refute what might be distorted theological explanations of suffering. Instead, we must cultivate acceptance of its mystery while we petition God for strength to persevere and await new hope to be born. In addition to cultivating acceptance of the mystery of suffering, the ill person and those caring for them should nurture reflection on sins in need of repentance and move toward a greater embrace of Christ's sacrificial death. A spiritual caregiver might encourage the ill person to read Psalm 32 or 51 and gently probe whether there is anything unconfessed weighing on the heart. Illness often prompts deep self-reflection that unearths sins in need of repentance. Hence, feelings of guilt that surface in illness can serve as an invitation to seek God's forgiveness. Dismissing guilt by simply saying that "God does not punish with illness," and not pursuing its source further, risks missing an opportunity to lead the person to the cross. Suffering, and the deeper self-reflection it forges, creates an opportunity to experience Christ's forgiveness and the Father's unconditional love in new and transformative ways. Even as our bodies fail, we can experience fresh spiritual life as we more deeply experience what the psalmist affirms, "As far as the east is from the west, so far does he remove our transgressions from us" (Ps. 103:12).

In Sharon's case, Sister Gloria knew that Sharon's past marked by sexual promiscuity and drug addiction had truly been forgiven, and that she had been transformed by the Spirit. She reframed Sharon's negative interpretation by directing her focus to Jesus's blood, the source of our redemption and forgiveness of sins. As Scripture says, "The blood of Jesus his Son cleanses us from all sin" (1 John 1:7). Even mature believers can fall into seeing God through a darkened lens, picturing him as Judge rather than the Lover of their souls. Spiritual care gently redirects these distorted impulses by reflecting on the cross. From the cross, Jesus makes clear that the harsh judgments we hear belong to the accuser of our souls, not to the Father (Ps. 31:15). For those who trust in Christ, God's hands are tender and protective, engraved with our names (Isa. 49:16; John 10:28–29). In those hands are all our days, both now and for all eternity.

Hope in the Healer

When facing pain or nearing death, we must fan into flame hope in God in the face of the temptation to lose hope. Whether as an ill person or as a caregiver, we are easily drawn to place our hope in medicine rather than in God, forgetting that all medical healing is enabled by God and only temporary. So while we are called to recognize and pursue medicine as good, we are simultaneously called to view all healing on earth as a dim foreshadowing of the resurrection to come. When properly understood, medicine points us to have hope only in God, the eternal Healer.

Whether navigating pain and suffering or feelings of divine judgment, the sick person must be continually led back to the cross, for it is at the cross where hope in our Savior is renewed. Jesus has fully cleansed us of our sins and justified us through his blood so that we can, with him, take up his final, hopeful words: "Father, into your hands I commit my spirit."

As part 2 has considered the words of Christ, we now turn to part 3 and our shared calling as a community. While illness and dying are deeply personal, they are never meant to be faced alone. Jesus's command in Matthew 25 to visit the sick is given not to a few specialists but to the entire community of faith. This section explores how congregations can walk together alongside the sick and dying. Organized around action, presence, and faith, these chapters show that caring well depends not only on what we do but also on how we are present and what we believe. Woven together, these commitments form a strong cord that supports the sick, sustains caregivers, and resists a death-denying culture. Together, these chapters describe a countercultural spirituality that lives out the words of Christ from the cross as we walk with one another on the journey home.

Part 3

Walking the Path Together

Eleven

Circle of Love

There is a time to cry
and a time to laugh.
There is a time to be sad
and a time to dance.
Ecclesiastes 3:4 NCV

We die best in community. . . . In fact, we might go so far as to say that it is impossible to die well if you die alone.

Lydia Dugdale

God's Circle of Love

"I want to bring everyone together," Lois said one morning, smiling and with her hands clasped as though in prayer. "Everyone who has been so beautiful and kind to me. I feel such deep gratitude. It is the love of God in me and through me. I want to thank God for giving me the strength to create something that honors this love. It is not just about me. It is about all of us. About community. About God's circle of love, light, prayer, dance, and roses."

She paused, catching her breath. "I am dedicating this service and dance to my Balboni family and to my church. I want to thank all the disciples who have cared for me during my illness. Melissa, Lisa, Ruth, Amy, Sarah, Joseph, Elaine, everyone who has prayed for me and fed me and kept me company when the nights were long. I have been surrounded by real disciples from God."

When Lois moved into our home, she was weak but still capable of moving small distances, such as navigating the stairs with assistance to join us for dinner. But each week she grew weaker. The walker soon became her partner, but then even that was insufficient as her body became more frail. Yet even as her body failed, her creative spirit flourished.

One evening, after a difficult day, she looked up and said, "I keep dreaming of a dance. A final dance. Not for performance but for praise. I want to call it 'God's Circle of Love.' It is not about death. It is about love that continues forever."

Lois had been a teacher and performer all her life. She had choreographed countless dances, designed costumes, and made props for theaters in Boston, Las Vegas, San Diego, and Barcelona. She had performed the Charleston and the Viennese waltz with the same grace that she once taught children in dance classes.

"Dancing is how I pray," she told us one night. "When I move, I am speaking with God. Before I begin a dance, I hold my partner's hand and whisper, 'Thank you, God. Thank you, Mom. Thank you, partner.'" Through this repeated prayer, she expressed gratitude first to God, then to her mother, who Lois believed gave her the gift of dance after she died, and finally to whoever shared the dance with her that night. "Dancing keeps me alive," she said.

Within a few weeks, Lois called everyone to begin coordinating "God's Circle of Love." As she planned and made phone calls, she sat up straight in her hospice bed, eyes bright, a notebook on her lap. "We are doing a dress rehearsal," she announced one day.

"This is not just a show. It is a symbol of community. It is about how we care for one another and how God surrounds us when we are weak." Everyone was assigned a part.

She arranged for us to rehearse at the church downtown. The challenge was getting her there. The stairs from our home to the car were difficult. "I will make it," she said firmly. "God will give me strength."

God indeed gave her the strength, and we were able to carry her into the car and drive into downtown Boston. When we rolled her wheelchair into the church hall, she looked around the room, smiled, and said, "This is perfect." Then, in an instant, she transformed from patient to director.

"I need everyone to listen carefully," she announced with confidence. She clearly had done this before.

"Michael," she said, pointing toward the front, "you will step in first, turning from your right to your left, counterclockwise. Then raise your left hand, palm up. Tracy, when Michael lifts his hand, you will touch it gently, twirl clockwise, and take your place in the circle. Each of you will follow, one after another, joining hands, forming a circle around me. Ten people forming one perfect circle."

We watched her, amazed. Every gesture mattered to her. Every step had meaning. "For me," she said quietly, "the nights have been lonely, and the road too long. But God has surrounded me with you. You are his circle of love and light. You are my strength. Now, let us begin."

For forty-five minutes, Lois directed us with the precision of a master choreographer. "Step with purpose," she said. "Lift your hand like you are offering it to heaven. Move slowly, breathe, feel God's love flowing through you." She planned to sit in the center of the circle, holding a basket of white roses. "When you come to me," she explained, "take the rose in your hand, bow slightly, and turn away slowly. Each rose is a gift of love, a symbol of how God turns mourning into dancing."

By the end of the rehearsal, we better understood Lois's vision, and what had sounded beyond odd to many of us now felt full of meaning. It was not a performance. Dance was symbolic of our entire spiritual community responding to and surrounding a friend in need.

Isolation and Community

Serious illness unleashes forces of separation and isolation. Being with others becomes difficult. Daily routines are disrupted, whether by physical limitations or by medical appointments, and work and other community responsibilities often end. Physical weakness and disfigurement can discourage social contact, making the sick less likely to attend social events such as weekly worship or to receive visitors. Ironically, people often grow in faith during illness yet find participation in religious life harder.[1] Family and friends may visit, but some withdraw out of discomfort, uncertainty, or lack of time. Illness cuts deeply into community connection.

Sometimes the sick self-isolate despite others' efforts to reach them. Illness can evoke alienation, regret, or fear. One pastor described a longtime church secretary who "locked herself in her hospital room and wouldn't allow anyone else to come in to see her. She spent most of her time weeping. It was a sad death." Another priest reflected, "I have seen people that were very isolated because of some of the choices they've lived. They had basically broken ties. . . . I think that is probably the worst." In such cases, anger and despair can harden into barriers that make care difficult.

God's intention is not isolation but healing within community. Wholeness is upheld and can deepen when the sick are surrounded by love and presence. Historian Guenter Risse describes a monastic vigil in which "some brethren remained with the dying inmate throughout the day and night, praying and reading from the Scriptures by candlelight. The point of this vigil was to ensure 'proper passing'; nobody should be left to die alone. If death became imminent, the whole monastic community was summoned and the monks congregated around the sick on both sides of the bed alternately to pray and sing, using music to 'unbind' the pain and thus provide the departing with spiritual nourishment for the journey to the beyond."[2]

Do communities still desire such vigils today? Many spiritual leaders say it remains central to community life. A Baptist pastor from Chicago's South Side said, "I firmly believe that we should be born into a community and we should die in a community." And a Roman Catholic priest in his seventies reflected, "A good death, I say a 'holy death,' will be surrounded by family and friends."

At its best, Christian community reflects the very nature of God. God's unity is a divine community—the Trinity—that is the essence and wellspring of love. The nature of this love is not inward, but rather inexorably outward as it seeks to receive those without a community of love. In Christ, God opens this community to the sinful, the stranger, the broken, and the sick. The divine community responds to sin and evil through divine action. This redemptive action reaches out to restore those consumed by the isolation of sin. While sin separates, divides, and draws people into darkness, divine community gathers, welcomes, communes, and brings into the light. The church in Christ is called to be a community like the Trinity—a community whose actions are energized by his love toward the broken, sick, and dying.

Lois was a beneficiary of an existing congregational ministry of care focused on people like her. Its purpose was never to replace family or close friends but to form a wider circle of care that could carry people through seasons of illness, grief, and crisis. The heart of the ministry was to listen first, discern real needs, and respond in ways that honored dignity and fostered relationship. Practical help was always paired with prayer, and care was offered with clear boundaries so that support felt steady, not overwhelming. Over time, those who served came to be known as "angels," not because of extraordinary deeds but because of their faithful presence and willingness to lift and shield those in need. At its core, the ministry reflected a belief that walking with others through hardship is a shared calling and that faith is lived out through coordinated acts of love, presence, and intercession.

For Lois, many such angels stepped forward. One helped her manage a car that kept breaking down. Several regularly drove her to medical appointments or sat with her in waiting rooms. Meals were brought a few times each week. After Lois received her diagnosis but before her first surgery, she could no longer afford her apartment, and a group from the church helped her move into subsidized housing. Others called to check in and pray or visited to read Scripture or a chapter from a book. One person brought her electronic piano, set it up in her room, and returned often to play it for her. A physical therapist volunteered time to help Lois retain strength for walking. Another brought her two young daughters to visit, knowing how much Lois loved being with children. Together, these angels did far more than complete tasks. They formed a circle of care that held Lois in prayer, relationship, and hope.

In such companionship, both the sick and their caregivers are transformed. As the suffering walk through the valley of shadows, the Good Shepherd provides fellow travelers for comfort and courage. Those who give care also receive gifts: Fear of death softens, life's brevity becomes clearer, and the wisdom of numbering our days deepens (Ps. 90:12). Within God's circle of love, all are changed, both those who receive care and those who offer it.

A good death is one surrounded by God's circle of love.

Integrative Church Support

Spiritual communities vary in how they provide care because they are shaped by theological and cultural influences.[3] According to

Susan Dunlap, such care may take practical, spiritual, or symbolic forms. Evangelical or Word-centered churches often emphasize practical action, charismatic communities prioritize spiritual engagement, and eucharistic traditions highlight symbolic expression. As Christian communities reflect on their particular tendencies, we recommend that churches seek to integrate all three approaches to create a more holistic ministry of care.

One model of caring for the sick centers on practical support and pastoral presence. Mainline Protestant, Reformed, and Evangelical churches often emphasize this approach. This model values patient dignity and privacy, trusts medical professionals, relies on community organization, and views illness as a test in which the community helps the sick endure and overcome.

Deacons or volunteers visit the sick, organize meal deliveries, offer transportation to medical appointments, and assist with household or childcare needs. Some congregations include volunteer or paid medical professionals who help members navigate complex health systems. Churches often maintain prayer chains or weekly prayer lists, sending cards and notes of encouragement. Pastors focus on spiritual care—helping the sick encounter Christ through emotional and faith-based support.

A second model described by Dunlap is oriented around the Holy Spirit.[4] Many charismatic and minority churches accentuate this method. Because of past medical injustices and limited medical access, these communities may distrust health care systems and can interpret illness as a spiritual battle in which healing comes through faith. Congregations pray, anoint with oil, and sometimes fast or intercede intensely for the sick, celebrating any healing as a testimony of divine power.

A third model, seen in sacramental traditions such as Roman Catholic and Eastern Orthodox churches, blends family, faith, and ritual. Care may include the anointing of the sick, home altars with candles and prayers, and masses offered on the sick person's behalf. Illness is surrounded with symbolic meaning and sustained communal presence.

In caring for Lois, our community wove together these three paradigms. Practical help surrounded her: she received rent assistance from the benevolence fund, deacons like Heather and Lisa drove her to appointments, and Tracy helped her wade through medical decisions. When Lois could no longer live independently, volunteers helped sort through her belongings, while others brought her favorite meals. During her stay in our home, she received daily visits from church friends. Our home was transformed into a living extension of the congregation's care. People learned to not bother knocking but just come in. Hailee, our golden retriever, was our official greeter, since we were often absent during the weekdays because of work.

In Lois's circle, many prayed fervently for a miracle early in her cancer diagnosis. After her final surgery, she entered hospice expecting to live only weeks, yet she survived eight months. During her inpatient hospice, our community anointed her with oil, sang hymns such as "Amazing Grace" and "Come Thou Fount," and prayed for healing. The singing drew in hospice staff; a nurse and cleaner, both Christians, joined in song to Lois's delight. "Pastor Michael," she said later, "you must meet Susan—she sings like an angel!" While prayers for healing were not being answered physically, we were witnessing aspects of Lois's healing emotionally and spiritually.

Lois's artistry and desire to connect self, community, and the transcendent inspired her not-yet-dead funeral. It was a service of love, light, dance, and roses. Her ritualized dance symbolized completion and unity within the community. It was a symbol that transformed her suffering through dance into white roses. Though she did not use the term *Eucharist*, it was profoundly sacramental as an outward sign of spiritual realities.

Each of these three paradigms found expression in Lois's care. Taken alone, each model of care only reflects a piece of who God is; together, they form a fuller theology and practice of community care and action. The practical model reveals Christ the Comforter, offering tangible help and counsel. The spiritual model proclaims Christ the Victor, uniting believers in faith and hope. The sacramental model embodies Christ the Suffering Servant, binding families through symbol and solidarity. In isolation, each approach risks slipping into stoic endurance, misplaced blame, or passive resignation. But when integrated together, they form a dynamic, holistic ministry of community care.

Evaluating Community Responses to the Sick

Every spiritual community has distinct strengths and weaknesses in how it responds to illness. Assessing and periodically reevaluating these patterns within your own community is vital to forming a more complete circle of God's love. What follows are rough generalities in care emphases by faith communities, with many exceptions; still, illuminating tendencies can aid in revealing where a fuller approach to the care of the sick is needed.

Mainline, Reformed, and Evangelical traditions often emphasize rationality and organization, qualities that readily meet ill persons' needs for practical help. However, they may also show hesitance toward healing prayer, anointing with oil, or healing expressed in liturgical symbolism. A rational approach can unintentionally minimize emotion, lament, or anger at illness and suffering. Some may avoid praying for miracles altogether. A more balanced model will include prayers for healing, symbolic acts such as anointing with oil (James 5:14), and public gatherings of prayer and thanksgiving.

Pentecostal, Holiness, and charismatic communities often emphasize prayerful intercession for healing, faithfully following

Jesus's call to heal the sick. However, they can also lean toward neglecting a theology of suffering or the call to endure illness with acceptance of our finitude. A more expansive approach would be to marry charismatic practice with practical and sacramental approaches to healing. When the Spirit does not heal, practices of lament, endurance, ongoing presence, and tangible service such as providing meals or transportation embody the Spirit's compassion.

Sacramental traditions offer profound rituals that bring reverence and hope, yet symbolic acts alone cannot replace consistent community presence with suffering or faith-filled intercession for healing intervention. Anointing and prayers should lead into companionship through the illness journey. Priests and lay leaders alike must carry hope not only in resurrection but also in the Spirit's present sustaining work. True pastoral care requires walking patiently beside the sick in both ritual and relationship.

Shepherds in Action

As spiritual leaders, pastors hold a pivotal role in the care of the seriously ill. On average they spend about four hours per week visiting the sick.[5] Pastoral theologian Thomas Oden aptly writes, "The flock is dispersed and scattered vulnerably about in a hazardous world. They will be shielded from thieves and led to fresh water only if the pastor is in the same field with them."[6] To this end, pastors have responsibilities in individualized care and visitation, as well as community-wide responses of vision-casting and organization.

Whenever a congregational member is seriously ill, it is incumbent for pastors to visit.[7] The visit by a pastor need not be long, but certain components will be included, depending on the patient and situation. As we will discuss in greater detail in the next chapter, spiritual care begins with asking questions and listening.

One pastor explained: "We have two ears and one mouth, so we must listen twice as much as we speak. In ministry, our task is to let people tell their stories again and again because they need to. When we truly listen, the moment for the spiritual response will come naturally." In a natural conversation grounded in presence, the pastoral visit may unearth unaddressed anxieties, fears, and spiritual questions. In such an engagement, the pastor might read an appropriate Scripture (sometimes arising in the mind by the Holy Spirit within the conversation). Sometimes there will be a discussion of a salient spiritual truth. The pastor may possibly offer the sacraments, and if granted permission, gently hold the patient's hand while offering a prayer of faith for healing in body, emotions, relationships, and soul. While every encounter varies, the pastor channels God's compassion, wisdom, hope, and presence. It is a unique and sacred encounter through which the Holy Spirit uses the office of pastor toward wholeness and certainty.[8]

However, visitation of the sick belongs to the entire community (Matt. 25:36), not just pastors. As a spiritual leader, a pastor is to teach, cast vision, and empower the community to organize so that all are encircled by God's love. As an older Texas pastor told us, "If it doesn't start with the pastor, then it really won't go to the congregation." Throughout the year, there should be teaching and stories on a theology of suffering, illness, dying, and hope in the afterlife. Lay persons are also to be trained and empowered to recognize material and spiritual needs. Lay persons can learn how to comfortably pray with the sick, share a Bible verse, and be authorized to bring communion to shut-ins and the seriously ill. The shepherding of the sick belongs to all.

Framework for Congregational Holistic Care of the Sick

The church's relative marginalization from caregiving with medicine's rise has resulted in the neglect of congregational frameworks for holistic care for the sick. Congregations and their leaders are encouraged to rebuild such frameworks, with prayerful attention to the ways the framework should be uniquely designed for each community setting. Holistic care for the sick involves practical, spiritual, and sacramental components, as shown in the framework below (see appendix B). Congregations are invited to adopt elements of each of these approaches to holistic caregiving; how each congregation chooses to manifest these components will be unique.

Practice-centered actions should enable practical care for ill persons and preparation for illness and dying for healthy congregants. Congregations should build care frameworks with congregational leaders (e.g., deacons and elders) and volunteers that ensure distribution of care responsibilities and the provision of needed resources (e.g., meals and rides) as they arise. Health care professionals within the congregation can be important resources by providing clinically informed guidance to care structures within the congregation.

Practice-centered actions should also include community preparation. Congregations should regularly discuss readiness for serious illness and dying and offer ways for members to prepare (as discussed in chap. 5). Such community conversations about end-of-life issues can help people confront and overcome death denial as well as facilitate key practical steps toward preparation. For example, congregants can be encouraged and taught how to create a legal will and assign a health care proxy. Prepurchasing a burial plot and prepaying for funeral services are also acts of personal responsibility that ease the burden on loved ones. Notably, based on the National Clergy Study, over one-third of clergy surveyed had not yet taken these steps themselves; congregational leaders are encouraged to do so in order to understand the process, model preparation, and provide for their own families.[9] Faith-based programs such as Here to Honor and secular organizations that intentionally include religious perspectives such as The Conversation Project and Five Wishes provide valuable frameworks for death education.[10] Additionally, Kathryn Butler's *Between Life and Death* is an excellent Christian resource for lay readers seeking to understand the medical care system and decisions encountered at the end of life.[11] Many congregations also have access to medical professionals, lawyers, and local hospice organizations who can help educate members directly.

Spirit- and sacrament-centered actions are also critical components to a holistic approach to care for the seriously ill, with examples provided in the framework in appendix B. These are best shaped by the unique communities and traditions, charisms, and callings of each particular faith community. Faith communities are encouraged to prayerfully consider practices to manifest the Spirit and to provide sacraments in the care of the sick, together with practice-centered approaches to caregiving. Such are opportunities for God's divine community to uniquely enter into the practical actions of love embodied by each congregation.

Dance, Prayer, Light, Roses

During the week after the rehearsal, Lois's energy rapidly faded. She had planned to attend the highly anticipated event in person, but on the morning of the gathering, she weakly whispered, "I cannot go. My body is too heavy. There is no way I can get out of bed."

We hesitated, unsure whether to go through with "God's Circle of Love." Lois took my (Michael's) hand. "Please, you still must do it," she said. "You must dance. God's circle does not depend on me. It is in all of us."

Eva, our teenage daughter, stayed home with Lois, and we set up a livestream so they could watch together in Lois's room. At the church, we placed her basket of roses on a stool in the center.

Tracy sang "The Rose" and played the guitar, accompanied by Ruth on piano. The final verse of Bette Midler's song was subtly but deliberately altered, replacing "the sun" with "God's Son" as the source of love that brings the rose to bloom out of the snows of winter.

When the song ended, the piano continued the melody. We followed Lois's instructions, forming the circle, lifting our hands, and moving together. And as we moved, the purpose behind the dance was embodied. It was a dance of faith, a circle of prayer, a community that had taken action, and in so doing we manifested God's divine community of love.

Each of us had stepped forward and picked one white rose from the basket. We then handed the remaining roses to everyone in attendance.

When the dance concluded, and with our roses in hand, the congregation said together with one loud voice, "We love you, Lois!" How funny that she wasn't watching from heaven but rather through Tracy's iPhone.

When we returned home, Lois was eagerly waiting and wanting to talk. We gathered as a family in her room.

"So," she asked, "how was the dance?"

"We followed every step, just as you showed us," Tracy said.

She nodded slowly. "Then I was there," she realized. "You see, this was always for God, and you are my circle."

She looked at each of us, her eyes shining.

"We belong to one another," she said. "That is what God wants us to remember. When one of us is weak, the others hold the circle. When one of us falls, the others lift us up. That's the circle of love."

Later that evening, as Michael went through the routine of putting Lois to bed, he read to her from the Gospel of John: "Truly, truly, I say to you, unless a grain of wheat falls into the earth and dies, it remains alone; but if it dies, it bears much fruit" (John 12:24).

We all experienced the truth of those words that day—within our odd little community dance, time and eternity touched. Lois, in her dying, taught us not only how to dance but also how to be a community of God's love. It is hands joined, hearts lifted, circling, twirling together within God's divine dance of love.

Twelve

A Community of Presence

Historically speaking, Christians have not had a "solution" to the problem of evil. Rather, they have had a community of care that has made it possible for them to absorb the destructive terror of evil that constantly threatens to destroy all human relations.

Stanley Hauerwas

The Lord's people will also enjoy light in *the hour of death*. Unbelief bemoans the evening shadows, the darkening night, the end of existence. But no, cries faith, the night is almost over and the true day is at hand. Farewell, loved one, you are gone. You wave your hand; now it is light! The pearly gates are open; the golden streets shine in the jasper light. We cover our eyes, but you behold the unseen; adieu, dear friend, you have light at evening time that we have not yet.

Charles Spurgeon

Undivided Presence

It was a warm midsummer Saturday. An unusual hush filled our normally bustling home. Tracy was traveling for work, the kids were off at camp, and for the first time in the six months that Lois lived with us, I (Michael) had an evening entirely alone with her. I did not recognize it then, but later I would see clearly that the Holy Spirit had ordered the night. Not one detail was accidental.

She had a few visitors earlier that day, but by late afternoon, the house was silent. I decided to prepare a simple meal for both of us: Boston baked beans and a fried hot dog in a toasted bun. I brought the plates into her room and with an exaggerated voice said, "Dinner is served."

Her smile appeared instantly. "Oh, Michael, you made my favorite. Thank you."

We ate slowly, with me on the couch and her in the hospice-provided adjustable bed. The rolling table and the commode on the opposite side of the bed had also been provided by the hospice agency. These were now necessary as Lois could no longer walk.

I had been working on my sermon for the next morning, and although I was trying not to show it, it didn't feel finished. After a moment she said, "Michael, you seem nervous about tomorrow. Will you practice your sermon with me? I want to hear it."

I smiled. "The whole thing?"

"Yes. Come on. It will help you."

So, after I cleared the dishes, I sat on the couch near her bed and began to preach through my sermon on Psalm 128, a Psalm of Ascents. I talked about fear and how it shapes us—fear of loss, rejection, failure, and death. I explained how fear can shrink a soul or twist it into domineering anger. I outlined the steps: name the fear, pray into the fear, and claim God's blessing over the fear.

Lois listened with great intensity. She stopped me several times. "Michael, maybe try another word there." And once she said, "You sound a little unsure. Slow down. Be calm and confident. You know this."

I laughed. "You're still the teacher, Lois."

"Well," she said, smiling, "someone has to keep the preacher grounded."

Her small edits helped, but then she fell quiet after I finished. Her eyes turned thoughtful. "This fear you're preaching about," she said carefully, "it has been pulling at me. I have been afraid of dying. But I have also been afraid of losing control of what little life I have left."

I could sense something more was on her mind. "Lois," I asked gently, "is there something you want to talk about?"

There was a long silence. The air felt charged, as though the Spirit had stilled the room.

"Yes," she whispered at last. "There is something. I need to tell you the truth about something."

I felt nervous but waited in silence. I tried to calmly smile, realizing that she was afraid. There was a long pause before she finally began speaking.

"I have not been honest with you about money," she said. "I have eighteen thousand dollars in savings. And last week I gave a large gift to a friend. I told you something else so that you wouldn't know."

I stayed quiet, letting her speak.

"You and Tracy have taken care of everything," she said, her voice trembling. "You've shown me unconditional love. But I was afraid. Money has always been a place of fear for me. I grew up poor, and it never left me. When I finally had enough to help someone, it felt important. But I hid it from you. I thought you might be upset if you knew I gave that gift while you were absorbing so many costs. And I wanted to keep control."

I finally said, "Lois, this sounds like it has been a big burden you have been carrying. I'm really grateful you told me. Can I ask you a question?"

"Yes, of course," she said.

"Why did you hide it from us? Haven't we shown you that we love you no matter what?"

"I know," she said. "You have been more than loving. But fear took over. If I could go back, I would have told you everything from the start. Will you please forgive me?"

I reached for her hand. "Of course I forgive you. Fear makes all of us hide. But you do not need to be afraid with us. And you never need to be afraid with God. Jesus said the truth sets us free. Tonight you are free."

She breathed out as though a giant weight had been lifted from her chest.

I asked, "Do you want to pray through the three steps from the sermon together?"

"Yes, Michael. That seems right."

And she prayed, "Dear Lord, I have been holding on to earthly things instead of releasing them to you. I was afraid to lose control. I confess that I sinned against you by letting fear grip my heart. Thank you for forgiving me. Thank you for Michael's kindness. You have blessed me more than I ever imagined. I have nothing to fear."

When she finished, the room was peaceful.

For a while we sat in quietness. Then, after a pause, I asked, "Lois, do you feel up to watching a little TV with me? I want to learn more about ballroom dancing."

Her eyes perked up. "Do you think you can find PBS's *Championship Ballroom Dancing*?"

"I don't know," I said. "I've never even heard of it."

"Well," she said, lifting her chin, "look for it."

Through search mode I found a rerun on cable. We agreed that we both needed a cup of ice cream.

Throughout the program she burst with excitement. "Look at that heel turn! Michael, do you see her frame? That is a perfect Viennese rotation. See their footwork? They are SO good."

I did not understand a thing. But as I watched I kept glancing at Lois. She came alive, narrating every technique. Her joy filled the room.

It was the perfect ending to a five-hour "date" that the Spirit had arranged.

The next day, Lois listened to me preach on the radio and later told our daughter, Eva, "Your dad preached a great sermon." No one knew, but she helped make it so.

By the time I came home that evening, Lois was sleeping. Tracy met me in the hallway. "Something is happening," she said quietly. "She is coming in and out of consciousness. I think she likely has brain metastases."

"What does that mean exactly?" I asked.

"With cancer growing in her brain, things can change quickly. She may die very soon," Tracy replied.

Only in the days that followed did the weight of our last night together come into focus.

It had been the Spirit's orchestration from start to finish. Lois's last supper, her last confession, her last forgiveness, her last dance. The Spirit made sure nothing remained unresolved.

Lois's last confession left us both unburdened. It was her final gift. And my final gift, despite the busyness of life and the demands of pastoring, was that I gave her my undivided presence on what would be her last night of full consciousness.

A Ministry of Presence

The church is called into a ministry of presence to the seriously ill and dying. A ministry of presence is the compassionate practice of being fully and attentively present with a suffering person. This includes listening, accompanying, and honoring the person's pace and needs without trying to fix, direct, or control the encounter—trusting that God is already present and at work.

While practical congregational actions are crucial (see chap. 11), equally important is the Christian community being available, listening, and being physically present. One Boston pastor described it this way: "Try to be present, not necessarily offering a whole lot of reasons for anything, but just supportive listening, encouraging. That is a role that the church and the congregation can play in the person's life who is facing terminal illness."

A theology of presence is rooted in the incarnation of Christ, who took on flesh, making himself immediately available and close (John 1:14). This divine event turns our focus from a God who acts and fixes toward a God who enters our lived experience. Presence recognizes that God is immanent, embedded in the fabric of the world. The Spirit is revealed in the good within each person made in God's image. The suffering person becomes a "living human document," their unique life a text of the Spirit's revelation to the community that is truly present.[1]

Presence in congregational care is the compassionate practice of being fully with the sick; staying relationally attuned rather than driven by ritual, agenda, or outcome; letting the sick lead the encounter; valuing simple human connection, including physical nearness; and listening and affirming emotion.

A ministry of presence is shaped not by what one does, such as performing sacraments or offering counsel, but by the quality of being with another. Rituals and words matter, but they cannot replace human relationship. One Catholic priest told us, "Presence is probably the greatest thing. . . . We tend to slip into, 'I anointed them so they don't need me anymore.'" A Methodist minister lamented visitors who aim to "preach to somebody who's dying," calling such an agenda "unforgivable" because it empties the relationship. Spiritual attunement meets the person where they are spiritually, emotionally, and existentially. The caregiver reflects the presence of Christ, who did not coerce but dwelled among us.

Allowing the sick to lead orients presence as patient-centered; it means releasing control and allowing the ill person to guide the encounter. Presence listens, follows, and honors the person's pace and needs. This form of ministry trusts that the Spirit is already at work. "Where shall I go from your Spirit?" asks the psalmist. "If I make my bed in Sheol, . . . even there your hand shall lead me, and your right hand shall hold me" (Ps. 139:7–8, 10). A pastor from Chicago's South Side described it this way, speaking from a neighborhood acquainted with loss and endurance: "You get into the muck with them, and you walk beside them. . . . It is a ministry where you need to allow the person to determine where you are going to go." A Boston clergyman said, "For the most part I let them direct the conversation. I don't go in with a goal and a purpose and intention. I follow their lead."

Trusting that the Spirit is already at work, the caregiver can wait for the person, and the flow of interaction, to reveal what matters. When the sick person raises a question or expresses emotion, it signals readiness. This approach requires calm courage to listen and to follow where the person is ready to go. When life is ending, pastoral care may need at times to be more direct, yet always within the bounds of relationship and the Spirit's timing, honoring the dignity of the one who suffers.

Some of the most sacred moments arise not from explicit spiritual talk but from simple listening, remembering, or sitting quietly with another in their vulnerability. One pastor reflected, "Here was this older woman in a lot of pain, discomfort, but you could see the joy of her reliving her life because I was just there with her and allowed her to talk about what she needed to talk about. So it [seemed to have] nothing to do with God, nothing to do with faith, and yet it did, as part of our humanness." Eating hot dogs and baked beans, watching a rerun of *Championship Ballroom Dancing*, and laughing together with Lois were moments of shared humanity that invited and mysteriously manifested God's presence. Presence is also offered through physical closeness and gestures that communicate humility, equality, and care. A hand held or a tender touch, where welcomed, offers comfort and reminds the sick they are not alone. A pastor who was also a part-time hospital chaplain shared, "I have found that if somebody is in the hospital, particularly someone who is dying . . . I kneel beside them so I'm looking at them eyeball to eyeball, as opposed to looking down at them [which creates] a sense of superiority." Such gestures affirm that human connection is sacred, expressing the spirit of Romans 12:15: "Rejoice with those who rejoice, weep with those who weep." In this way, the grace of God is revealed in our common humanity.

Harmful Presence

In the book of Job, we find a remarkable account of three friends who travel from afar to comfort Job in his suffering. For the first seven days, they sit in the dirt with him in silence. It is a beautiful gesture of presence and lament, and we can imagine that Job took comfort in their sacrificial gesture and simply from not being alone. But everything soured the moment they began to speak. Their shift from silent presence to speech led to misspoken words, harsh judgments, and additional suffering for Job.

Their failure is a timeless warning when ministering to the sick or suffering. It is easy to speak rashly, to say the wrong thing, or to attempt to fix what cannot be fixed. So we must be admonished by their example and pray that the words of our mouths offer grace, not harm.

The classic mistake shown by Job's friends is to say or even imply that illness is the sick person's fault. Such statements are not only inaccurate; they are often a psychological means for the speaker to protect themselves from discomfort or fear—if suffering is interpreted as a consequence of a person's actions, then one feels less vulnerable to the same fate. One church member shared how his resentment toward a former pastor began when that pastor visited his dying mother. During the visit, the pastor suggested that her illness persisted because she lacked faith, implying that unanswered prayers were her fault. Those words devastated her. Her son tried to console her, but she felt condemned and hopeless. This experience left a lasting conviction in him that such words are not only wrong, they are cruel.

In Luke 13, referring to eighteen people who perished in a tower's collapse, Jesus admonishes us not to cast judgment as to who is more or less deserving of a calamity. Another mistake occurs when we enter a sickroom with spiritual agendas that reflect our own internal needs rather than the needs of the person. Those who are seriously ill are vulnerable and weary. If we step into a room with our own agendas rather than walking in step with the Spirit, we are likely to fail to bring comfort and can even risk harm. We have been blessed to witness beautiful and genuine deathbed conversions, but these were ultimately the work of the Holy Spirit. We should pray into the possibility for spiritual breakthrough and growth, but we must be attentive to and follow the lead of the Spirit as we interact with an ill person. Spiritual care is about walking the sick home, not dragging or coercing them.

When we visit someone who is sick, we often feel pressure to say something comforting. Silence can feel awkward, and we may worry that saying nothing means we do not care. But in that pressure, it is easy to speak too quickly or reach for familiar phrases that can end up hurting rather than helping.[2] For example, with the intent to foster connection, we might say, "I know what you're going through," or "When I went through that . . ." As well intentioned as such words may be, we can't assume our own experience is the same, and that assumption could actually be minimizing to that person's suffering. Furthermore, we must also be careful not to focus on our own experience. There is no absolute rule as the Spirit surely wants us to draw from our own suffering, and perhaps at certain unique moments to make mention of our suffering is appropriate. Yet the overwhelming primary focus should always be on the sick person, not the one who is visiting.

We might offer quick reassurance: "Everything is going to be okay," "God will get you through this," or "I'm sure things will turn out well." These statements can sound hopeful, but they make promises we have no right to make. None of us knows the outcome.

Sometimes we try to lighten the moment with comparison: "At least you have . . ." or "At least it's not . . ." Yet those phrases, while attempting to express gratitude or perspective, can minimize the person's real suffering.

Other well-intentioned sayings come from Scripture but can be spoken too hastily: "All things work together for good," "God won't give you more than you can handle," "Everything happens for a reason," or "God must be teaching you something." While these are biblical truths, we need to be wary of selecting truths based on our own needs for explanation or simply for words to say. Scripture reading is a central aspect of ministry to the sick, but we need to be listening to the person and attentive to the Spirit to recognize what are helpful, timely words for the sufferer to hear.

It is far better to ask questions, listen more than you talk, and allow silence to hold space for compassion. Often, quiet presence and a few sincere words of prayer communicate far more love than any well-meant but hollow declaration.

Our calling to care for the sick is not to explain their suffering, fix their situation, or fill the silence. It is to be present, to bear witness with gentleness, humility, and prayer. Sometimes the holiest ministry we can offer is the ministry of quiet presence.

Presence Through Questions

Empathic or active listening is the art of being fully attentive, compassionate, and understanding. This is one of the greatest gifts we can offer. As James reminds us, "Be quick to listen, slow to speak" (1:19 NIV). By learning to listen well, we pattern ourselves after God. While presence is fostered through empathic listening, it is deepened through open-ended questions. Throughout the Bible, we find God asking questions in difficult moments. "Where are you?" (Gen. 3:9) he says to begin a conversation with Adam and Eve after they have sinned. When the prophet Elijah hides in fear, God asks, "What are you doing here, Elijah?" (1 Kings 19:9). After Peter's three denials, Jesus asks him, "Do you love me?" (John 21:17). Of course, God already knows the answers to the questions. He knows the thoughts and motives of every heart (Ps. 139:2). His questions are meant for the hearer; they invite transparency and self-examination within relationship. The one who is asked is dignified by being allowed to respond without presumption. And in responding, the person is invited into a greater awareness of themselves and a deeper relationship with God.

When experiencing suffering, our tendency is to lash out in frustration and anger toward God, ourselves, and others. Illness is evil, and anger toward evil is an appropriate response. However, in our humanity, we can misdirect that anger. Even Job, who was righteous before God, misspoke from within his pain. God knew Job's heart perfectly, but he confronted him by asking questions, beginning with, "Who is this that darkens counsel by words without knowledge?" (Job 38:2). Job responded to his friends' accusations with his own misspoken words and false accusations toward God. God, in his patience, love, and desire for Job's spiritual growth, probes him again with a series of questions. God's queries reveal how Job's suffering has led him to wrong conclusions and ultimately bring him to a deeper understanding and relationship with God. Job concludes, "I had heard of you by the hearing of the ear, but now my eye sees you" (42:5).

For those visiting the sick, our questions should intend to help the sick person deepen self-understanding and grow in their relationship with God. There are broadly five categories of spiritual challenges within serious illness: meaning, identity, faith, relationship, and hope. These deal with the basic matters of existence, and they are not merely theoretical but deeply personal to the person facing illness and death.

If you are visiting a sick person with whom there is a relationship or connection, asking questions that encourage exploration of possible spiritual challenges within illness can be beneficial. Let's walk through example questions a patient might have in these five areas, followed by questions that the caregiver or listener can respond with to deepen the conversation:

1. Questions of Meaning: How do I fit into this world? How is my life a part of the bigger picture?
   - Looking back, what are the moments of your life that are especially important and meaningful to you?
   - As you look at your life now, what do you think really matters?
2. Questions of Identity: Who am I when I have nothing left? Who am I without my job/kids/health?
   - Since your illness began, has your sense of who you are changed?
   - Has the illness in any way stripped away any false sense of self? Do you see more of who you really are at the core, regardless of being healthy or sick?
3. Questions of Faith: Where is God? What is my relationship to God?

- How have you experienced God's presence and absence during this time?
- How would you describe your relationship with God right now?
- Have you experienced God speaking or showing you new things in this time?

4. Questions of Relationship: Who do I need to thank? How do I mend this relationship?
    - Are there any relationships on your heart? People you want to reach out to or things you need to say to someone?
    - Is there any person you need to forgive or from whom you need to ask forgiveness?
    - Do you have any life regrets you'd like to talk about?
5. Questions of Hope: What do I have to look forward to? What can I be hopeful about?
    - For however many days you have remaining, is there anything undone that you think you should try to finish or accomplish?
    - As you look beyond death, do you have hope?

How to Practice Listening

Drawing upon both medical and pastoral experience, the ministry of presence can be understood as a journey. The movements below as you enter a person's space can guide pastors and laypersons in many settings, whether at home, in hospitals, or in nursing facilities.

At the Threshold

Before entering, pause for a moment and take a slow breath. Offer a short prayer: *Lord, let me see Christ in this person; let me offer you to this person.* Ask the Holy Spirit to calm your heart and help you let go of the day's distractions. This visit is not about having perfect words or fixing anything. It is about offering Christ's presence. Anyone can be present, not only professionals. Enter with a peaceful spirit, soft tone, and open heart. A calm visitor can change the atmosphere of a room.

At the Bedside

Greet the person warmly and by name. Introduce yourself if needed. Notice how they are doing and respond with simple kindness: "It's good to see you today. Thank you for letting me stop by." A gentle handshake, when appropriate, can affirm dignity in a situation that may feel far from normal. Sit at or below eye level as a posture of humility that communicates, "I am here with you." Allow silence if words feel heavy. Sometimes a quiet presence says enough.

In the Quiet Spaces

Listen with your whole self. Empathic listening means paying attention not only to their words but also to the feelings and fears beneath. Let the person speak at their own pace. When you stop worrying about what to say next, listening becomes more natural and free-flowing. Reflect back what you hear: "It sounds like this has been really hard." "I understand why you want to go home." "Of course you're concerned for your children." Avoid quick explanations or clichés. Naming and validating emotions often brings relief to the sick and the sense that they are understood.

As the Conversation Deepens

When someone feels truly heard, they may naturally open to deeper questions of meaning, faith, and hope. If the moment feels right, you might say, "What helps you keep going right now?" "How have you been experiencing God during this illness?" or

"What gives you hope these days?" Do not press for responses. Silence after such questions is normal. In the quiet, pray inwardly and wait. Listening itself often helps people discover what God is stirring within them. You are not there to interpret their suffering but to create space where faith and doubt can both be spoken openly.

At the Point of Connection

After listening, respond with compassion by briefly acknowledging what you've heard: "You've been through so much, and it's remarkable to hear your story marked by so much strength." "This diagnosis is overwhelming, yet I hear hope in your voice." If it feels appropriate, offer prayer: "If it would be helpful, I can pray for you before I go." Sometimes extending your open hand may lead the person to hold it, which can bring comfort to someone feeling isolated. Keep the prayer simple. Do not use prayer to preach. When it is time to leave, thank them: "It has been good to visit with you. May God's peace be with you."

Guarding Trust

Confidentiality is essential. If the person shares something that may need to be communicated to the pastor or others, ask permission: "Would it be all right if I shared this with the pastor?" or "Do I have your permission to share this prayer request?" If permission is not obtained, the information should be kept private. Trust is easily broken and hard to rebuild.

On the Way Out

After you leave the room, pause for a moment to reflect and pray. Acknowledge what you experienced, including any sadness or heaviness. This helps guard against burnout. If a visit goes poorly, seek support promptly with a person who can provide wisdom and experience. At times, we may unintentionally give offense; at other times, those who are suffering may respond with unkindness. Difficult encounters should be considered carefully and prayed through with a trusted, experienced church leader. We all need support in these moments. Being around deep suffering can be emotionally weighty, so set healthy boundaries for yourself. In prayer, release the person you visited into God's care. This is an important reminder that we are companions in ministry, not the ones who carry the full burden. Ask God to hold what you have heard and to renew your spirit as you continue the work of caring.

Empathic listening is simple in principle, yet it calls for humility and steady practice. As you grow more comfortable, you will find it easier to ask thoughtful questions and to sit quietly without feeling the need to fill the silence. It requires letting go of the urge to fix, explain, or advise and instead to offer a calm and loving presence. When you enter a visit with attentive ears and a compassionate heart, the space becomes holy ground. In listening, we join the Holy Spirit in his quiet work, drawing near both to the patient and to God. Most moments will feel ordinary, but there are times when you may sense that God's Spirit is moving in the room and through one another. When that grace reveals itself, it is a cherished gift. We must remember, though, that we cannot expect to see the full spiritual impact of our care for the sick in Christ. Just as the early Christians who cared for abandoned children and plague victims did not see the fullness of their work until they joined the great cloud of witnesses in heaven, we likewise are yet to see the fullness of our work in him.

Walking Lois Home

On July 27, 2021, I (Tracy) wrote an email to our church family, trying to put words around what was unfolding in our home. I sat at my desk and typed, "Michael and I wanted to update you all about our dear sister, Lois, and ask for your continued prayers as she enters the final leg of her journey on this earth." Even as I wrote those words, the truth pressed on my heart. Lois was dying, and we were preparing ourselves for the sacred task of walking her all the way home.

Six months earlier, the Lord had brought Lois into our lives with such unexpected grace. Those months were full of laughter, her digital artwork, her creativity, her bold visions of dance, "God's Circle of Love," prayers for our church, and prayers for us. She grew in faith right before our eyes. She fully surrendered her life to Christ. She was baptized in her hospice bed. She prayed nightly with us. She often told me she was ready for the Lord to take her home.

But a few days before I wrote that email, her medical condition began to shift. She developed some neurological symptoms suggesting cancer had spread to her brain, including becoming intermittently confused and then increasingly somnolent. She was lucid on Saturday, when she had spent the evening with Michael. She was even able to listen to Michael's sermon on the radio on Sunday morning. But then through the rest of that day she became increasingly confused and required greater medications for headaches and nausea. She went to sleep early that evening. On Monday morning, I could barely awaken her for her medications. I called the hospice agency to let them know. That was when Michael and I realized we were beginning a vigil—one we would hold until the end.

"She cannot be alone anymore," I told Michael.

"Okay," he answered, "how are we going to do this?"

From that moment on, one of us was beside her day and night. Others from our church helped so we could take breaks. I moved my oncology work to a room immediately across from Lois's room, where she was always in view and I could check on her frequently, which was only possible because COVID restrictions had moved most of my medical practice to the virtual setting. At night, Michael and I traded shifts. One of us would sleep on her couch until early in the morning when we would trade roles. Our presence was the one thing we could still give to her.

Hospice intensified their visits. Nurses came twice a day, sometimes for an hour. They cared for her meticulously and administered pain medications so she remained peaceful. Changing her incontinence briefs at night was physically challenging. After the hospice nurse left in the afternoon, the task would fall to us. Thankfully our dear neighbors Felix and Melanie came over to help. Felix, a surgeon by training, and Melanie, a nurse practitioner, were familiar with this kind of care. Melanie guided us through every step. I remember standing beside them that first night, rolling Lois gently, lifting her carefully.

"Lois," I whispered, "Felix and Melanie are here. You have met them before. They are helping us take care of you."

Even though her eyes were closed and she could not respond, we could sense her discomfort. Though she was not conscious, we explained everything to her, step by step. Felix spoke gently, "Lois, we are going to move you a little now. Just to keep you comfortable." Melanie, given her nursing background, knew exactly how to move, clean, and reposition her.

There was something strangely sacred in caring for her, even though it was physically demanding addressing such basic needs. The four of us surrounded her with reverence. At the end of one of those changings, two nights before she died, Lois had a moment of near-consciousness and reached her hand weakly for Michael's. As Michael grasped her hand, she said in the faintest whisper, "I am lucky." They were the last words she spoke.

In the intensity of those days, we did not understand her reference. We recognized it only afterward. It was a soft echo from the song I sang as part of our dance "God's Circle of Love." The lyrics of her favorite song refer to "the lucky" as the ones who experience love in its fullness in this life. Lois in her nearly inaudible words was sharing her experience of Divine Love—love that was carrying her through the winter and "bitter snows" of this life. Two days later, on July 30, 2021, the end came.

That morning, I relieved Michael at 4:30. I lay on the couch beside her, barely sleeping because her breathing had become uneven and labored. I rose every few minutes to check on her. Around 6:15 a.m., I finally got up and sat beside her with a Bible someone from church had left. Three passages were marked: Psalm 30, Psalm 63, and Psalm 149. All spoke of praising and dancing with the Lord.

I touched her hand. "Lois," I said softly, "someone marked these for you. I am going to read them to you now."

> You have turned for me my mourning into dancing;
>   you have loosed my sackcloth
>   and clothed me with gladness. (Ps. 30:11)
>
>   My mouth will praise you with joyful lips,
> when I remember you upon my bed,
>   and meditate on you in the watches of the night;
> for you have been my help,
>   and in the shadow of your wings I will sing for joy.
> My soul clings to you;
>   your right hand upholds me. (Ps. 63:5–8)
>
> Let them praise his name with dancing,
>   making melody to him with tambourine and lyre!
>   (Ps. 149:3)

I read each psalm aloud as a prayer. Then I sang one of her favorite hymns—one we had sung many times together before—"When I Survey the Wondrous Cross." As I sang quietly over her,

her breathing shifted. It slowed. Then slowed again. The end was near.

> Were the whole realm of nature mine,
> that were an offering far too small.
> Love so amazing, so divine,
> demands my soul, my life, my all.

I leaned close to her. "Lois, I am right here," I whispered.

I then called for Michael, who had just awoken. He rushed from the third floor and stood beside me at her bedside. Lois's breath was now gone.

The morning light poured into her room. It was seven o'clock.

Michael and I prayed over her together. "Lord, receive your daughter. Your precious daughter."

Lois was now with God.

At her bedside was a printed prayer that had been given to her by her father years earlier. After his death she carefully placed it in an elegant frame, and she kept it at her bedside as a quiet reminder of him. Beneath the prayer, written in her own hand, were the words "For my father, George Frederick Meinhardt Sr. 1888–1985." Michael and I, together with our church community, had the privilege of journeying with Lois through the final months of her life, and through death, as this prayer was surely fulfilled:

> A Prayer of Gratitude
>
> *Loving and gracious God, my help in the past, source of my present strength, and my hope for the future, accept my gratitude for being with me during my days of difficulty and transition. Thank you for being my help when helpless, my strength when weak, my hope in despair, my light in darkness, my guide in confusion, my comfort in distress, my savior when lost.*

Thank you, too, for the hope and assurance of life's eternal nature and that death is not the end of life. It is not like the period at the end of a sentence but like a comma—marking a transition into a new and different form of life where we continue to live with you and in the hearts and minds of loved ones and friends. Continue to be with me, and eventually may I sense anew your peace that passes all understanding. Amen.

Thirteen

Dancing with Lois

You have turned for me my mourning into dancing;
you have loosed my sackcloth
and clothed me with gladness,
that my glory may sing your praise and not be silent.
O LORD my God, I will give thanks to you forever!
Psalm 30:11–12

When I met my first dance partner, I challenged him to the
Charleston swing—music played and we began our dance.
That's when everyone started to watch, so I took a chance—
I pulled away, but he followed me.
He said, "I've never danced with anyone that can do what
you do,
you followed me and I followed you."
So—follow your passion and create your stage identity,
It binds you to the audience and to your partner.
They can't teach you what you have, they don't have the
nerve.
People feel it and they love it. You're a born entertainer.
And it's indescribable, the energy of her dance.

Like she was shot out of a cannon, dancing the can-can.
So—go out and feel the passion of the moment,
And dance!

a poem by Lois Meinhardt, dated May 27, 2021,
which she left for us to find after her death

A Comma, Not a Period

The first time we both met Lois in person was in October 2020, after Lois's cancer was found to have spread and was considered incurable. After learning of this development in her cancer diagnosis from her oncologist, she called Michael, sounding desperate. She was upset and confused. After that conversation, we decided to both visit her at her apartment. I (Michael) wanted Tracy to come along with the hope that she could help Lois with her medical knowledge.

We arrived wearing masks—it was the middle of the COVID-19 pandemic. Gusts of wind blew off the ocean under heavy gray clouds. The uneasy atmosphere matched the weight of the moment. When we stepped inside, Lois immediately voiced her fear. "These medical people are so confusing. I do not understand a thing they are saying. They use all these strange words. I think I'm dying."

She looked up at Tracy and asked, "Am I dying?"

Tracy answered calmly, "That is not a simple question. There is a chance that surgery and radiation could control the cancer for a time. It is not curable, but with treatment you could live for a few more years."

Lois became visibly less tense as Tracy explained what was happening and why treatment was still a good option.

We had brought supper from a local pizzeria. As we ate pizza and talked, her emotions settled, though she remained serious.

As our conversation came to a close, I asked, "Lois, would you be willing to share what you believe about death? What do you think will happen after you die?"

"I have thought about this a lot," she replied. "I want to show you something my father gave me." She stepped into her bedroom and returned with a small, decorated frame. "He gave me this years ago. I love this line." She read it aloud slowly and with feeling. "Death is not like the period at the end of a sentence but like a comma—marking a transition into a new and different form of life."

She looked at us and said, "Pastor Michael, that is what I believe about death. It is not the end. It is a comma marking new life."

Our walk with Lois through her journey with serious illness was never about convincing her of eternal life. She already believed, having adopted the trusted wisdom of her father. Rather, it was about helping her move through fear so she could actively live into that belief. As it turned out, this season also challenged us, along with many others, to become more of a community of faithful believing.

From that shared pizza supper forward, we would not only be walking Lois home. She would be teaching our entire community how to dance—how to live with faith and belief in the life God brings after death.

Community of Believing

The church is invited to live out its Christian call to love the sick and dying in our actions (chap. 11), in our presence (chap. 12), and lastly, in our faith and beliefs (chap. 13). In this chapter, we will explore how the church can faithfully live out its belief that death does not have the last word.

In the aftermath of death, there are powerful emotions and ongoing grief, yet Christ has given Christians resources that offer guidance and hope. These beliefs and practices are rooted in the immortality of the soul, hope in the resurrection of the body, the importance of lament, and a commitment to the communion of saints that binds together the living and the dead.

Together, these Christian convictions and practices shape how the community remains connected to those who are dying and how it cares for the body after death. They shape the funeral and guide the ways healing can unfold throughout the long journey of grief. The church is called to be a believing community that walks through death together, trusting that communion and meaning do not end but continue and grow.

Grief

As soon as Lois died, we felt a complex set of emotions including sadness and relief. Our sadness stemmed from the obvious rupture of relationship. Love creates a bond between persons in which our minds, bodies, and identities are intertwined. Death severs these ties, resulting in an immense divide (Luke 16:26). The dead are shrouded behind a veil, a barrier like the ancient veil of the Holy of Holies, where the living cannot enter and cannot see what lies beyond. In addition to this loss of connection, there is a disruption of meaning. Death challenges the identity of those left behind. It raises questions of why, and after the initial shock, grief challenges the bereaved about their own future in light of such loss.

Depending on many factors, grief is experienced in waves, and for certain people, it may take a long time to learn to live again. The bereaved often face exhaustion, sleep disruption, and physical manifestations such as chest tightness, gastrointestinal distress, and heaviness in the body. Grief triggers a roller coaster of emotions, including intense sadness, anger, guilt, and numbness. Bereavement often makes it difficult to concentrate, leads to intrusive thoughts, and results in replaying memories and what-ifs. Connecting with God may become difficult. Death sends shockwaves as the realization of the loss of love and meaning is gradually absorbed.

Grief is a highly individual experience, dependent on personality and personal history, relationship, culture, and the circumstances surrounding the person's death. For some, grief takes months; for others, years. Not infrequently, some get stuck in their processing of grief, requiring pastoral check-ins, possibly professional counseling, and support groups such as GriefShare.[1]

Other emotions arise too. For example, we felt sadness but also relief when Lois died. We knew she was no longer suffering, including from pain and from the losses caused by her illness. We were also relieved to no longer be under the heavy burden of caregiving. It was physically and emotionally exhausting to care for Lois, particularly toward the end of her life.

Even with support from hospice and from surrounding community, the burden falls especially on those who are tasked with medical decision-making and with the daily chores of caregiving. Our relief when Lois died at first felt strange or even wrong in light of the sadness of death. But upon further reflection, we recognized that Lois was better off—she was free of suffering and was with God. We also more fully appreciated the heavy burden of caregiving after it was removed and we could return to a normal life routine. The caregiving burden can be so consuming that the caregiver can forget what life was like without the caregiving role. For some, the sudden loss of caregiving can be disorienting. Providing care can be so all-encompassing, it can define one's identity. Caregiving takes a major toll on caregivers, certainly in the form of time and energy but also in the complexity of emotions that attend caregiving both during care and after the death of a loved one.

Despair and Tragedy

Although Lois's death was deeply sorrowful, it was anticipated and thus carried less of the weight of tragedy. Most deaths are "mixed" in their nature; they include aspects of resolution but also incompleteness.[2] A death is "mixed" or more tragic when marked by suddenness, unpredictability, violence, or injustice. It can also arise when a person dies in profound isolation, doubt, or despair—when meaning appears lost or hope out of reach.

We do not believe it is theologically or pastorally helpful to interpret a person's state near death as reflective of their spiritual state before God. Several pastors we interviewed emphasized that a person's last words, their mental health, or the despair they may feel near the end do not determine their fate after death. While we hope no one faces tragic or unresolved moments in dying, many deaths include unfinished or painful elements. For example, we learned later that Lois had an estranged sibling (she called herself an only child, but later referred to a "brother," perhaps a half brother or stepbrother). She had not communicated with him for many years, and this relationship remained unresolved at the time of her death. This reflects the idea of death as a comma rather than a period. For most, some matters will be left unresolved. Of course, we hope for and encourage reconciliation and resolution before death where feasible, but even when these beautiful moments occur, they are only signposts of the full restoration found in God. Finally, we are admonished as followers of Jesus to eschew all judgments of others, and that is certainly the case in death. "There is only one lawgiver and judge, he who is able to save and to destroy. But who are you to judge your neighbor?" (James 4:12). Instead, the church should work to foster a community that surrounds those who face dying with assurance of forgiveness through Christ's atoning blood and with hope in the beautiful life to come.

Controversial forms of dying that are becoming more common are physician-assisted suicide (PAS) and euthanasia.[3] In our national survey of clergy, most remained morally opposed.[4] Such practices violate the sacredness of the divine image and fail to surround those who suffer with a community of love and presence.

The church is called to prepare one another for death (chap. 5), accept finitude (chap. 8), and relieve pain in every way we can (chap. 10). We are to accept death as the last enemy (1 Cor. 15:26) when it comes, not to purposely or willingly cause it.

Additionally, as a number of bioethicists have argued, PAS and euthanasia place implicit and coercive pressure on the elderly, the disabled, those with cognitive decline, and those suffering severe depression.[5] When vulnerability is seen as a burden, death begins to appear as relief for both the sufferer and those around them. And as bioethicists Curlin and Tollefsen have argued, involving physicians in decisions that intentionally end life also threatens the trust at the heart of the medical vocation, whose purpose is to heal and to comfort, not to kill.[6]

These challenges also present an opportunity for the church to live into Christ's calling. It is inadequate to solely criticize laws legalizing PAS without also stepping forward as communities marked by action, presence, and faith. Those who are most vulnerable need Christian communities willing to draw near in love. If the church truly lived out the command of Jesus to visit the sick and surround the dying with his compassion, would this not be a powerful witness to dignity and hope?

Mixed and tragic deaths will remain part of a broken world until Christ returns, yet the Christian community can still bear witness to the love of God and to hope in the life to come, even in tragedy. When we stay close to those who suffer, refusing to abandon them and offering compassionate presence, many of the fears that lead people to consider ending their lives are eased. Lois nearly ended her life, and we remain grateful that we answered her phone call and entered her pain. How great the harm would have been for her and for us if the church had failed to be the church. What would have been lost had she pursued such a path? When Christian communities give in to such despair, the consequences are far greater.

Loss and Gain

Scripture speaks with a kind of double vision about death. It is both foe and friend, both an intruder upon God's good world and, at the same time, a doorway into the presence of Christ. King Hezekiah's lament in Isaiah 38 captures the first truth. He is young, heirless, and facing national crisis; nothing in his life feels complete. His grief is not a failure of faith but an honest naming of reality. Death is a rupture and an assault on God's common grace. Scripture never asks us to disguise this. It teaches us to mourn, name the breaking of relational bonds, and feel the knife that death drives into human love and meaning.

Death is a real loss, and it is right to say so. As Hezekiah reminds us, "The living, the living—they praise you" (Isa. 38:19 NIV), and this is precisely what makes death grievous: It cuts short praise that belongs to God. Death silences worship. Thus, Scripture teaches lament. Lament is the honest cry of mourning, weeping, and longing voiced throughout the Psalms. Psalm 13 captures this powerfully as David repeats his agonized question, "How long, O LORD?" (v. 1). The Psalms are filled with pointed questions back to God: Where? (Ps. 89:49). Why? (Ps. 42:9). How long? About 40 percent of the Psalter gives voice to this protest. As discussed in chapter 4, Jesus himself prayed a lament from the cross (Ps. 22:1; Matt. 27:46). Even God's own posture toward suffering is described in the language of grief: The Lord laments over Moab (Isa. 16:9–11), over the fall of his people (Isa. 22:4), and over the nations in their ruin (Jer. 9:17–19; 48:31–32). In this way, lament becomes a faithful acknowledgment that death interrupts the praise of the living.

Yet against the shrill tone of lament, the church also believes Scripture's call to eternal life.[7] When a believer dies, the spirit is immediately welcomed into the presence of God. The faithful are described as "the spirits of the righteous made perfect" whose names are "enrolled in heaven" and who in death are "living" (Heb. 12:22–23; Matt. 22:32). Jesus promises the repentant thief, "Today you will be with me in paradise" (Luke 23:43), and Paul speaks of death as "to depart and be with Christ, for that is far better" (Phil. 1:23). The souls of the faithful therefore rest by the altar of God in conscious blessedness as they communicate directly with the Lord (Rev. 6:9–11), for "the spirit returns to God who gave it" (Eccles. 12:7), while they await the final resurrection when "the dead in Christ will rise" (1 Thess. 4:16) and our bodies will be "raised imperishable" (1 Cor. 15:52). And no matter whether we call this reality the intermediate state, sleep, paradise, heaven, or Abraham's bosom, the point is that those in Christ gain an immediate and fuller presence to the divine. We lament, but in their state after death, we can perhaps say that they are more alive than the living. As C. S. Lewis creatively imagined, the living are more like ghosts, whereas the redeemed become truly solid, entering into "an eternal weight of glory beyond all comparison" (2 Cor. 4:17).[8]

As an example, Tracy had a patient who was in her twenties, Mary, whom she met early in the course of her metastatic cancer. Tracy prayed and hoped for her miraculous healing, burdened by the sadness of the tragedy of this beautiful young woman's illness. When all treatments failed, Mary opted for hospice care. Tracy said goodbye to her in the hospital and, following the Spirit's prompting, gave her a bracelet she was wearing with a tiny inscription paraphrasing Psalm 46:5: "God is within her. She will not fall." Mary left the hospital to be cared for by her family at home, and Tracy did not hear from them for several weeks. Then one early morning, Tracy awoke from a vivid dream about Mary. In the dream, Tracy was going to visit Mary in the same hospital room where she had last seen her and given her the bracelet. Just as she was about to open the door to the hospital room, Mary burst through the door, strikingly radiant and wearing garments beyond words with their beauty. Beholding her, Tracy realized,

"She is more alive than I am." Upon awakening, Tracy immediately thought that Mary must have died. Indeed, only a few hours later, Mary's family let her know that she had died that same morning. Tracy, with some trepidation, shared the dream with the family. They were amazed and asked if she might share the story at Mary's memorial service. And so Tracy shared this story of hope—of a future life that renders all in this life a mere shadow in comparison—in the midst of sadness and tragedy. At the conclusion of the service, Mary's mother brought the bracelet, saying that Mary had treasured it and worn it until the moment she died. God was indeed with Mary; he did not let her fall. The concluding words of Psalm 46:5 seem prophetic upon reflection, as Mary burst into newness of glorious life at the "break of day" (NIV). This is the hope we are called to embrace and proclaim as a community of God, even in the face of tragedy and death.

This hope does not erase but reshapes sorrow. We do not grieve "as others do who have no hope" (1 Thess. 4:13), because we trust that the believer who dies has entered a deeper fellowship with Christ, one awaiting its completion at the resurrection of the dead (1 Cor. 15:52). One day our redeemed souls will be rejoined to newly raised-up physical bodies. Death becomes not a defeat but a transition to a new beginning. Thus, the two truths stand together without contradiction. Death is loss, and we mourn it. Death is gain, and we trust God as we face it. For those who die in Christ, living does not end. Death is no longer *It*; rather, death is a portal, an expansion of the praise of God begun in this life, yet continuing in a fullness that is better by far (Phil. 1:23).

When we walk with those who are grieving the death of someone who did not have faith or did not live well, we must speak carefully, honestly, and with deep compassion. The Christian hope of heaven and final judgment can bring a measure of comfort, especially in a world where great injustices often go unanswered. At the same time, Scripture reminds us that being welcomed into God's presence is not earned by being a good person but is grounded in the love of God and the saving work of Christ. Again as C. S. Lewis helpfully taught, God is not a distant judge who reluctantly lets people into heaven.[9] God is love, and he welcomes all. Yet God does not force himself on anyone. Hell, whatever its mystery, is best understood not as God delighting in punishment but as the tragic outcome of a life that finally refuses God's presence. In this sense, God gives people what they have chosen: life apart from him. We also trust that God judges each person with perfect justice, holding them accountable only for the light they have received. Jesus himself taught that greater revelation brings greater responsibility (Matt. 11:20–22). In the end, every person rests in the hands of a loving and just God, and his hands are where we place our trust. We do not know the final state of another's soul, and we are not called to decide it. Our comfort is that God will do what is right, merciful, and good. The most important question is not where another stands before God but how we ourselves are responding to his grace.

Commendation and Commitment

Eternal life continues to be in tension with a culture of death denial, not only during serious illness but also in the sacred tasks of care and love involved after death. Thomas Long has written that Christian rituals of burial grew from a believing community that gathered to worship in accompanying the dead with prayer and hope.[10] A Christian burial is not shaped merely by a need for the therapeutic or celebrating life or managing grief, though these are essential matters of the heart. When made primary concerns, these impulses often reflect a culture uncomfortable with death. For example, Long offers criticism of services that "celebrate life," not because celebration is improper but because such services tend to mute grief as everyone tries to keep the tenor positive. The deeper Christian instinct is to gather with faith in the promise of resurrection, even as we acknowledge that death has severed bonds of love and disrupted our sense of meaning.

A community of faith believes that the body matters. The person's postmortem body is sacred and central to their future. To lay a body to rest is not to discard something useless but to return a gift to the earth in trust. Scripture describes the body as a seed sown in weakness that God will raise in glory. It is more than a cadaver that decomposes. It is the embodied self that the Spirit will one day transform. As Paul teaches, the body that is sown is not the body that will be, for God gives it a new and greater form that we cannot yet fully imagine (1 Cor. 15:38). When death disrupts our relationships and confuses our story, our community of belief holds to this promise of transformation.

This raises practical questions about burial and cremation that deserve careful, pastoral reflection. Christians have historically practiced burial, placing the body in the ground. This most closely follows the pattern of Jesus, who was laid in a tomb (John 19:41–42). Time and nature return the body to the earth. As a practice, burial is intended to express tenderness and care, as nothing is done to hasten decomposition. The ground is set apart as sacred, enabling loved ones and future generations a place to remember those who have gone before.

A primary concern is not about the method of disposition but about practices that minimize ritual, memory, and communal care. Some Christians also understandably experience a symbolic tension between cremation and biblical images of fire and judgment, not as a biblical prohibition but as a matter of meaning and imagination shaped by Scripture.

These concerns do not mean that cremation is inconsistent with Christian faith when practiced with reverence and intention. Helpful guidance can be found in Roman Catholic teaching such as the *Ad resurgendum cum Christo* from 2016, which reflects

Christian instincts shared across traditions.[11] It teaches that when a body is cremated, the remains should be placed in a dedicated and reverent location where loved ones and the church can gather to remember and pray. For this reason, some hold that ashes are best not scattered, kept privately, or divided, not out of a critical spirit but because the body belongs to God and is held in trust by the whole Christian community.

These practical considerations aside, our eternal hope is not determined by how remains are handled. Many families make these choices out of love and grief. Still, whenever possible, the church is called to serve as a faithful custodian of the body, offering visible signs that even in death, we belong to God and to one another.

This also reflects the ancient Christian approach that funerals echo baptism. As Paul says, "For if we have been united with him in a death like his, we shall certainly be united with him in a resurrection like his" (Rom. 6:5). Our gathering around the dead person and laying their remains into the ground reflects the theology of baptism, in which the believer is buried in Christ with anticipation of being raised again.

One central act of the funeral liturgy is the sending away of the body in commendation and commitment. The Book of Common Prayer (1928) says, "Unto Almighty God we commend the soul of our [brother or sister] departed." To commend is to release the person's soul into the hands of God, as Jesus did when he prayed, "Father, into thy hands I commend my spirit" (Luke 23:46 KJV). In commendation, the community lets go and entrusts the whole person to God's keeping. To commit is to entrust the physical body to its earthly resting place, as the community's direct handling of that body ends. Again, familiar words: "And we commit [his or her] body to the ground; earth to earth, ashes to ashes, dust to dust; in sure and certain hope of the Resurrection unto eternal life, through our Lord Jesus Christ." The commitment of the body to God is a communal act of faith that what is or shall become dust will be made like the heavenly Christ (1 Cor. 15:48–49).

The funeral is a last collective act a believing community offers on its journey with the departing person. These ritual actions honor the person, body and soul. They acknowledge a shift in relationship. The one we love is not erased or simply gone but now rests in Christ and awaits the day of resurrection. We bless them in their going, we lament our sad separation, and we ask the Spirit to help us discover meaning. Yet there is faith despite no tangible resolution. Resurrection and reunion will come, and so even at the grave we sing songs, accompanying the departed on their journey home, entrusting them to our Lord who promises to clothe the perishable with the imperishable (1 Cor. 15:54).

Communion and Meaning

The church embraces the communion of saints named in the Apostles' Creed, and this belief shapes the way Christians walk through death and grief. The doctrine teaches that those who have died in Christ remain united with the people of God. Though their earthly life has ended and they have passed beyond death, the Holy Spirit holds us together in union with Christ. Reformers, such as Calvin, taught that the departed do not return to take part in daily life, a view most Protestants continue to hold, which helps guard this teaching from misunderstanding.[12] However, Scripture points to those who have died in Christ being mysteriously present to those of us living, such as the "great . . . cloud of witnesses" Paul describes as surrounding believers in Hebrews 12:1. This communion of saints is a fellowship that death cannot break.

Those who are with God now are held in his care, while the church on earth worships in weakness and hope. Even so, on both sides of death, we belong to the same redeemed family. Many Christians also understand this communion as pointing toward the full gathering of God's people when all things are made new. This provides clarification to Paul's words "that you may not grieve as others do who have no hope" (1 Thess. 4:13). Our grief is real, but it is not hopeless, because our life in Christ continues to bind us to those who have died in him.

This shared hope shapes the Christian approach to grief. It teaches that love between the living and the dead continues as a bond in Christ.[13] This view differs from the belief that holding on to someone who has died is unhealthy. A pastor can help grieving church members recognize that their sense of connection is not a failure to move forward. Rather, it is part of the fellowship God maintains. A pastor might gently say, "It makes sense that you still feel connected. They are with Jesus, and we are all mysteriously connected through him. Will you tell me more about how their life is strengthening and guiding you now?" In addition to affirming that connection in Christ, we can share our own sense of connection with a departed friend. For example, a church member might call a widower to say, "I was thinking about your wife today. Her kindness encouraged me. She helped me during a hard time. I miss her." This kind of remembering and holding connection beyond the grave demonstrates that love and connection can continue in healthy ways. In grieving together, there is a sense of validation and healing that is more difficult to experience alone.

The whole church joins in this work of healing. Through prayer, Scripture, and shared stories, the congregation should help mourners let the relationship take on a new and hopeful form. The church remembers the dead in worship, walks with the grieving in daily life, listens to stories when people are ready, marks important dates, and supports connections that honor the person's life. Many churches read the names of the faithful departed on All Saints' Day as a sign that their place in the congregation endures. Some churches keep a columbarium for members' ashes, which gives families a quiet place to remember loved ones close to the daily life of the church. In all these acts, the church declares that death does not erase the bonds Christ creates. Instead, God holds those bonds within his eternal life.

Grief is also a search for meaning.[14] Loss interrupts the story of our lives and leaves us unsure of who we are or where we are going. Healing does not come by forgetting the dead. It comes as we learn how this loss now fits within our story and how God may be shaping a new chapter. The communion of saints reminds us that those who have died in Christ still belong to us. Their love and witness can still guide us as we move forward. Meaning-making helps us ask how the person who died still shapes our life in Christ and what God may be calling us to next.

Lament is an important part of this process. Minister Mark Vroegop writes that lament gives us individual and corporate words to speak our pain to God, which enables healing by maintaining honest connection with God, rather than yielding to denial or despair.[15] Through lament, we remember what we have lost and also what has been received. Strangely, lament of the dead reveals what love continues to impart within us.[16] The gifts, values, and wisdom of the person who died remain alive in us through lament. Churches can support this work by creating times for shared lament and prayer. These moments often help new meaning and direction to arise in the hearts of the grieving. Death imparts gifts to the living, first experienced in lament, which in time can be carried into the next chapters of life. A pastor might ask those grieving, "What part of your loved one's life still calls to you?" or "Has this loss shown you new things or what matters most?"

Meaning-making does not rest only on individuals. It belongs to the whole congregation. For example, a member might say, "She showed me how important it is to care for international students. I want to continue that work. I wonder if others will join me? I believe she would want this." When a church wonders, prays, and acts together in writing a new chapter, the communion of saints becomes a lived reality. New meaning rises within the whole community. God brings healing and renewed purpose to all, often through the witness of those who have passed beyond the veil.

Walking Home as a Community

Our death-denying culture has quietly shaped the way Christians understand serious illness and dying, often leaving the church uncertain, avoidant, or overly reliant on either miracles or medicine. Modern medicine's material focus and the church's narrowed theology of healing have weakened Christian care for the sick. Too often, believers seek abundance only in this life, struggle to speak honestly about death, or cling to false hopes that prevent faithful preparation. But the church is called to recover a deeper and more balanced vision of love: one that acknowledges suffering, names fear, and refuses denial while trusting God's presence even in silence.

At the heart of this vision are the last words of Jesus on the cross. They shape a Christian approach that makes room for prayer for physical healing while also recognizing that healing may come in other forms, such as through repentance, reconciliation, and peace at the end of life. And all earthly healings are but signposts of the fullness of healing that comes by way of death in Christ and his resurrection. We've seen how illness strips away false securities and presses the soul to ask who we are when everything else is taken. In that refining fire, both the sick and those who love them are invited to discover the suffering Christ who meets us in weakness and leads us toward what is imperishable and eternal.

The care of the seriously ill belongs to the whole Christian community. When one member suffers, all are affected, and the Spirit forms the church into a collective of action, presence, and faith in foundational beliefs about eternal life. This includes practical help, attentive listening, prayer, sacraments, and the steady hope of resurrection life.

To be the church is to walk people home—not alone but together. We resist despair while speaking truthfully about death and holding fast to life beyond it. Living out our Christian call to love the sick and dying means reclaiming this shared work so that no one is unseen, unheard, or abandoned as they near the end, and so that the church once again bears faithful witness in the face of death.

Lois Ann Meinhardt, 1948–2021

Less than two hours after Lois passed beyond the veil, the hospice nurse arrived to care for her body. She asked for Lois's favorite dress. The nurse gently washed her and brushed her hair, and then Tracy and the nurse clothed her in her yellow dress and white cardigan. Her hands were folded tenderly. Lois's spirit was with the Lord, but her earthly body was still ours to honor.

Lois had long said she wanted to be cremated and to have her ashes placed at the shoreline outside her childhood home in Winthrop, next to the Boston Harbor. She loved her parents, her first home, and the ocean, and she believed this was the most fitting place for her body to await resurrection. It was the same location she had laid her parents' remains to rest.

For months she had spoken of gathering all her friends for a boat cruise and dance on the harbor. "I want us to do an afternoon cruise on the watah," she would say, in her thick Boston accent. "It'll be such a delight to have everyone together. The ocean is so mysterious and calming." Then, with her certainty and ingenuity: "Michael, I called an old friend who owes me a favor. He does boat cruises for groups up to a hundred people. I've scheduled a Saturday in June. I want to teach people the Charleston Swing right on the harbor. They'll never forget it!"

But as spring turned to summer, she grew too sick to make the dream possible. Teaching ballroom dancing was out of reach, and even getting out of bed became difficult. "I think I'll get better," she strained to say. "I really want to bring us all together."

A few weeks before the event, Michael told her reluctantly, "Lois, I know this is important to you, and I really want to do the dance cruise. But I'm worried that it may not be realistic."

"I know," she admitted. "You're right for now. Maybe I'll start to feel stronger, and then we can do it."

The next day, she called to cancel the boat and asked friends to release the date. It was a small but painful letting go.

After her death, though, we knew we needed to follow her instructions. On September 7, 2021, about a dozen of us gathered by the water. The afternoon was warm, and the sky deep blue. Friends shared stories, laughter rising as someone imitated one of Lois's dramatic twirls. Several lifelong friends and former dance partners came, including a few who, as often happens, had not even known that she had been sick.

Her childhood home stood just across the street. White shells adorned the sand like an arrangement she might have made herself. Across the bay, boats rested quietly, and a faint bell carried over the water. It was hard to imagine a more fitting scene.

Michael offered a few final words, remembering Lois as a woman of faith, an artist, and a dancer who faced death with courage. He read the psalm marked in her Bible: "You have turned for me my mourning into dancing; you have loosed my sackcloth and clothed me with gladness" (30:11). And then, in the sure and certain hope of the resurrection to eternal life through our Lord Jesus Christ, he commended her to God's care and committed her body to his mercy: earth to earth, ashes to ashes, dust to dust.

Two of Lois's closest lifelong friends carried her ashes to the edge of the shoreline, near the quiet marsh grasses, and returned her to the place where her parents rested. One day that body will dance again, even as her soul dances now.

Afterward we ate together at a restaurant on the harbor. Friends shared stories we had never heard. A childhood friend from church, after hearing that Lois had been baptized, exclaimed, "Praise God. I can't believe it. Knowing Lois, I never thought she would come back to faith." They all marveled how over the past year Lois had overcome her debilitating anxiety and faced down her fears.

In the end, Lois's wish—the one she had to surrender—came true in essence. Her friends gathered at the ocean. There was laughter and even a little dancing. And in a way she could not have planned, she taught many of us not ballroom dancing but a far more difficult and beautiful dance around illness and death. Caring for Lois became more than witnessing a beautiful sister in Christ twirling and leaping over her own comma. It became a new beginning for our community, rising to dance to the resounding music of Christ's call to love the sick and dying.

Acknowledgments

We are fortunate to work with our book agent, Janet Grant, who read and offered edits and important suggestions on several chapters in the book. We are grateful to Allisyn Ma and Rachel Welcher from Baker Books, who provided insightful suggestions and editorial support in the writing process. We are indeed grateful to the entire Baker team, who have provided incredible support, some of whom include Sarah Gordon, Carrie Weston, Robin VanderWall, and Julie Davis.

Nancy Bradley provided helpful feedback on early chapters and recommendations on persons to interview. We are deeply appreciative to the many individuals who gave of their time and wisdom as they were interviewed as part of this project.

We owe special thanks to our academic colleagues at the Harvard Initiative on Health, Spirituality, and Religion, including John Peteet, Tyler VanderWeele, Howard Koh, David Rosmarin, Laura Tuach, Katelyn Long, and Constantine Psimopoulos. It has been our privilege to work with them, not only as respected scholars but also as friends. We have also benefited from the wider scholarly community at Harvard, including support Michael received from the Human Flourishing Program at Harvard.

We are especially grateful to our congregation, Restoration Fellowship in Boston, for generously providing Michael with time for writing. Michael is especially grateful to co-pastor alongside a team of pastors and lay leaders who reflect the love and sacrificial example of Jesus.

Finally, we are deeply grateful to the many unnamed people who sacrificially loved Lois through their care.

Appendix A

End-of-Life Planning Checklist

Spiritual Preparation

- ☐ Ask God for wisdom and foresight, as well as energy and joy, in planning for your death.
- ☐ Invite a pastor to talk through spiritual matters in your relationship with God.
- ☐ Prayerfully consider how God may be leading you to offer blessings and bring closure to practical affairs and personal relationships.

Legal and Practical Planning

- ☐ Hire a lawyer or use online software to create a legal will, trust, and power of attorney. Complete and sign all paperwork, witnessed by a notary.
- ☐ Clarify and explain your estate plans to family members or others to avoid misunderstandings or disputes after death.

- ☐ Make funeral or burial plans so loved ones are not left guessing about your wishes.
- ☐ Organize important information such as financial accounts, passwords, insurance papers, and documents loved ones will need.

Medical and End-of-Life Decisions

- ☐ Establish a health care proxy and complete the legal document.
- ☐ Present the health care proxy document to your physician, proxy, and family members.
- ☐ Talk with your proxy about your goals. Discuss preferences for medical interventions in terminal illness, coma, or dementia.
- ☐ Discuss your wishes with your doctor so your goals of care are known and followed.

Relational and Community Support

- ☐ Identify a medical professional at church who may be willing to advise you when needed.
- ☐ Share your decisions with close family, friends, and caregiving partners so everyone understands your wishes.

Appendix B

Framework for Congregations to Provide Holistic Community Care for the Sick

Practice-Centered Actions: ***Practical, hands-on forms of preparation and care for those facing illness and death***

- Equip deacons and surrounding care teams with training, structures, and resources to enable practical helps (e.g., rides to appointments, meals).
- Include in sermons two to three times per year topics on suffering, dying, and the afterlife.
- Enable community discussions on death preparations (Here to Honor, The Conversation Project, Five Wishes; see chap. 11, note 10).
- Utilize congregational nurses, physicians, and lawyers for end-of-life education.
- Encourage pastors to personally complete legal and medical documents to enable awareness of practical processes and modeling of preparation.

Spirit-Centered Actions: ***Spirit-centered practices to invite and cultivate the Spirit's presence in the care for the sick***

- Provide Scripture readings (the "sword of the Spirit," Eph. 6:17) and prayers that those visiting the ill person can use, inviting the Holy Spirit to work in the ill person's, and their caregiver's, mind, body, and spirit.
- Hold a healing service with petitions for God's healing and work through sickness.
- Invite community prayer for the sick, including by posting the ill person's prayer needs (with permission) and by community prayer for the sick as part of services.
- Provide community space for testimony about and thanksgiving for healing of body, mind, and spirit.

Sacrament-Centered Actions: ***Sacred practices that uphold and provide symbolic expression of scriptural truths, such as Christ's presence within suffering, his atonement for sin, and the promise of full restoration in the life to come***

- Train and send eucharistic ministers to bring communion to those homebound and hospitalized.
- Create altars for prayers by lighting candles or lifting up the name of the sick.
- Train and send community leaders to anoint and pray over the sick.
- Provide sacred visual or other artistic elements to ill persons and their caregivers, such as a crucifix, sacred artwork, or sacred music.

Notes

Chapter 1 Introduction

1. Gary B. Ferngren, *Medicine and Health Care in Early Christianity* (Johns Hopkins University Press, 2009).

2. Eusebius of Caesaria, *The Church History of Eusebius*, in *Eusebius: Church History, Life of Constantine the Great, and Oration in Praise of Constantine*, ed. P. Schaff and H. Wace, trans. A. C. McGiffert (Eerdmans, 1952), 362–63.

3. We commend the writings of historian Gary Ferngren, who shows how Jesus and the Christian community transformed the meaning of illness, the practice of medicine, and social responsibility to care for the sick. See Ferngren, *Medicine and Health Care in Early Christianity*; Gary B. Ferngren, *Medicine and Religion: A Historical Introduction* (Johns Hopkins University Press, 2014).

4. For a more detailed discussion of this passage, see Michael J. Balboni and Tracy A. Balboni, *Hostility to Hospitality: Spirituality and Professional Socialization within Medicine* (Oxford University Press, 2019), 151–53.

5. Guenter B. Risse, *Mending Bodies, Saving Souls: A History of Hospitals* (Oxford University Press, 1999).

6. The English words "hospital," "hospice," "hospitality," and "host" come from the Latin *hosti*, which references "the stranger." The Latin root *pit* literally refers to "a feeder of" guests. Hence, "a feeder of strangers" can refer to the receiving of pilgrims, or the care of sick strangers.

7. "Oral History Interview with Cicely Saunders," August 11, 1993, John C. Liebeskind History of Pain Collection, https://www.iasp-pain.org/wp-content/uploads/2023/06/final_saunders.pdf.

8. In New Testament Greek, the term *astheneō*, typically translated "the sick," refers to someone burdened with various types of physical weaknesses, including disabilities, chronic illness, frailty due to old age, and dying. Accordingly, throughout the book we employ the biblical term "the sick" and "illness" to refer to a broad spectrum of physical weaknesses, each of which we are called to

care for. While most of the stories are with cancer patients, the principles and concepts are widely applicable across a range of chronic and debilitating illnesses, terminal diseases, and dementias.

9. We will primarily focus on evidence gathered through the empirical sciences in research conducted by us. We will focus on databases including the National Institutes of Health–funded Coping with Cancer Study, the National Clergy Project on End-of-Life Care, and the Systematic Review of Spirituality in Serious Illness and Health. The research we discuss in the book has been previously published in many peer-reviewed scientific medical journals. See especially: M. J. Balboni et al., "U.S. Clergy Religious Values and Relationships to End-of-Life Discussions and Care," *Journal of Pain and Symptom Management* 53, no. 6 (June 2017), https://doi.org/10.1016/j.jpainsymman.2016.12.346; T. A. Balboni et al., "Spirituality in Serious Illness and Health," *JAMA* 328, no. 2 (July 12, 2022), https://doi.org/10.1001/jama.2022.11086.

10. Balboni and Balboni, *Hostility to Hospitality*.

Chapter 2 ***It***

1. J. W. Mack et al., "End-of-Life Care Discussions Among Patients with Advanced Cancer: A Cohort Study," *Annals of Internal Medicine* 156, no. 3 (February 7, 2012), https://doi.org/10.7326/0003-4819-156-3-201202070-00008.

2. W. Slort et al., "Perceived Barriers and Facilitators for General Practitioner-Patient Communication in Palliative Care: A Systematic Review," *Palliative Medicine* 25, no. 6 (September 2011), https://doi.org/10.1177/0269216310395987.

3. E. Knauft et al., "Barriers and Facilitators to End-of-Life Care Communication for Patients with COPD," *Chest* 127, no. 6 (June 2005), https://doi.org/10.1378/chest.127.6.2188.

4. C. H. Chen, S. C. Kuo, and S. T. Tang, "Current Status of Accurate Prognostic Awareness in Advanced/Terminally Ill Cancer Patients: Systematic Review and Meta-Regression Analysis," *Palliative Medicine* 31, no. 5 (May 2017), https://doi.org/10.1177/0269216316663976.

5. Lydia S. Dugdale, *The Lost Art of Dying: Reviving Forgotten Wisdom* (HarperOne, 2020).

6. Aleksandr Solzhenitsyn, *Cancer Ward* (Farrar, Straus and Giroux, 1969), 100.

7. Philippe Ariès, *Western Attitudes Toward Death: From the Middle Ages to the Present*, Johns Hopkins Symposia in Comparative History (Johns Hopkins University Press, 1974).

8. In addition to Lydia Dugdale's work, Allen Verhey describes, critiques, and reimagines the tradition of the art of dying in his important theological reflections. Allen Verhey, *The Christian Art of Dying: Learning from Jesus* (Eerdmans, 2011).

9. This is called the "existential security thesis" argued by Pippa Norris and Ronald Inglehart, *Sacred and Secular: Religion and Politics Worldwide*, 2nd ed., Cambridge Studies in Social Theory, Religion and Politics (Cambridge University Press, 2011).

10. See S. H. Cross and H. J. Warraich, "Changes in the Place of Death in the United States," *New England Journal of Medicine* 381, no. 24 (December 12, 2019), https://doi.org/10.1056/NEJMc1911892; G. B. Risse and M. J. Balboni,

"Shifting Hospital-Hospice Boundaries: Historical Perspectives on the Institutional Care of the Dying," *American Journal of Hospice and Palliative Medicine* 30, no. 4 (June 2013), https://doi.org/10.1177/1049909112452336.

11. A. Kleinman, "Culture, Bereavement, and Psychiatry," *Lancet* 379, no. 9816 (February 18, 2012), https://doi.org/10.1016/s0140-6736(12)60258-x.

12. Ariès, *Western Attitudes Toward Death*, 91.

13. For example, Lecretius described how humans make incredible efforts to secure themselves against death by seeking greatness, status, importance, possessions, friendship, and pleasure (*De rerum natura*, 3.31–116).

14. Ernest Becker, *The Denial of Death* (Free Press, 1973).

15. Charles Taylor, *A Secular Age* (Belknap Press of Harvard University Press, 2007).

16. Agency for Healthcare Research and Quality, "Substance Use Disorders," in *2022 National Healthcare Quality and Disparities Report*, https://www.ncbi.nlm.nih.gov/books/NBK587182/; Merianne Rose Spencer, Arialdi M. Miniño, and Margaret Warner, "Drug Overdose Deaths in the United States, 2001–2021," NCHS Data Brief No. 457, December 2022, https://www.cdc.gov/nchs/data/databriefs/db457.pdf; Lauren J. Tanz et al., "Drug Overdose Deaths Among Persons Aged 10–19 Years—United States, July 2019–December 2021," *Morbidity and Mortality Weekly Report* 71, no. 50 (December 16, 2022): 1576–82, https://www.cdc.gov/mmwr/volumes/71/wr/mm7150a2.htm.

17. Haim G. Ginott, *Between Parent and Teenager* (Macmillan, 1969).

18. J. S. Vigdal and K. K. Bronnick, "A Systematic Review of 'Helicopter Parenting' and Its Relationship with Anxiety and Depression," *Frontiers in Psychology* 13 (2022), https://doi.org/10.3389/fpsyg.2022.872981.

19. R. L. Coley, J. Leer, and L. Lanteri, "Trends in Mental and Behavioral Health Risks in Adolescents: 1999–2021," *Pediatrics* 155, no. 4 (April 1, 2025), https://doi.org/10.1542/peds.2024-068774.

20. Kenneth I. Pargament, *Spiritually Integrated Psychotherapy: Understanding and Addressing the Sacred* (Guilford Press, 2007).

Chapter 3 Religious Denial

1. G. True et al., "Treatment Preferences and Advance Care Planning at End of Life: The Role of Ethnicity and Spiritual Coping in Cancer Patients," *Annals of Behavioral Medicine* 30, no. 2 (October 2005), https://doi.org/10.1207/s15324796abm3002_10.

2. T. A. Balboni et al., "Religiousness and Spiritual Support Among Advanced Cancer Patients and Associations with End-of-Life Treatment Preferences and Quality of Life," *Journal of Clinical Oncology* 25, no. 5 (February 10, 2007), https://doi.org/10.1200/JCO.2006.07.9046.

3. A. C. Phelps et al., "Religious Coping and Use of Intensive Life-Prolonging Care Near Death in Patients with Advanced Cancer," *JAMA* 301, no. 11 (March 18, 2009), https://doi.org/10.1001/jama.2009.341.

4. H. H. Bulow et al., "Are Religion and Religiosity Important to End-of-Life Decisions and Patient Autonomy in the ICU? The Ethicatt Study," *Intensive Care Medicine* 38, no. 7 (July 2012), https://doi.org/10.1007/s00134-012-2554-8.

5. H. S. Lam et al., "Attitudes Toward Neonatal Intensive Care Treatment of Preterm Infants with a High Risk of Developing Long-Term Disabilities," *Pediatrics* 123, no. 6 (June 2009), https://doi.org/10.1542/peds.2008-2061.

6. Michael J. Balboni and John R. Peteet, *Spirituality and Religion Within the Culture of Medicine: From Evidence to Practice* (Oxford University Press, 2017).

7. M. J. Balboni et al., "U.S. Clergy Religious Values and Relationships to End-of-Life Discussions and Care," *Journal of Pain and Symptom Management* 53, no. 6 (June 2017), https://doi.org/10.1016/j.jpainsymman.2016.12.346.

8. T. A. Balboni et al., "Provision of Spiritual Support to Patients with Advanced Cancer by Religious Communities and Associations with Medical Care at the End of Life," *JAMA Internal Medicine* 173, no. 12 (June 24, 2013), https://doi.org/10.1001/jamainternmed.2013.903.

9. Balboni et al., "Provision of Spiritual Support to Patients."

10. V. T. LeBaron et al., "Clergy Views on a Good Versus a Poor Death: Ministry to the Terminally Ill," *Journal of Palliative Medicine* 18, no. 12 (December 2015), https://doi.org/10.1089/jpm.2015.0176.

11. R. Hatch et al., "Anxiety, Depression and Post Traumatic Stress Disorder after Critical Illness: A UK-Wide Prospective Cohort Study," *Critical Care* 22, no. 1 (November 23, 2018), https://doi.org/10.1186/s13054-018-2223-6.

12. T. Amass et al., "Stress-Related Disorders of Family Members of Patients Admitted to the Intensive Care Unit with COVID-19," *JAMA Internal Medicine* 182, no. 6 (June 1, 2022), https://doi.org/10.1001/jamainternmed.2022.1118.

13. Kate Bowler, *Blessed: A History of the American Prosperity Gospel* (Oxford University Press, 2013).

Chapter 4 The Silence of God

1. See Kenneth I. Pargament and Julie J. Exline, *Working with Spiritual Struggles in Psychotherapy: From Research to Practice* (Guilford Press, 2022).

2. S. R. Alcorn et al., "'If God Wanted Me Yesterday, I Wouldn't Be Here Today': Religious and Spiritual Themes in Patients' Experiences of Advanced Cancer," *Journal of Palliative Medicine* 13, no. 5 (May 2010), https://doi.org/10.1089/jpm.2009.0343.

3. John of the Cross, *John of the Cross: Selected Writings*, trans. K. Kavanaugh (Paulist Press, 1987), book 2, chap. 5.

4. W. D. Winkelman et al., "The Relationship of Spiritual Concerns to the Quality of Life of Advanced Cancer Patients: Preliminary Findings," *Journal of Palliative Medicine* 14, no. 9 (September 2011), https://doi.org/10.1089/jpm.2010.0536.

5. Winkelman et al., "Relationship of Spiritual Concerns"; A. Damen et al., "Prevalence, Predictors and Correlates of Religious and Spiritual Struggles in Palliative Cancer Patients," *Journal of Pain and Symptom Management* 62, no. 3 (September 2021), https://doi.org/10.1016/j.jpainsymman.2021.04.024; F. Nazam and A. Husain, "Hope, Meaning in Life and Religious/Spiritual Struggle Predicts the Quality of Life in Cancer Patients with Early and Advanced Malignancy: A Structural Equation Modeling Approach," *Health Psychology and Behavioral Medicine* 12, no. 1 (2024), https://doi.org/10.1080/21642850.2024.2351936; M. J. Pearce et al., "Unmet Spiritual Care Needs Impact Emotional and Spiritual

Well-Being in Advanced Cancer Patients," *Supportive Care in Cancer* 20, no. 10 (October 2012), https://doi.org/10.1007/s00520-011-1335-1.

6. Pargament and Exline, *Working with Spiritual Struggles in Psychotherapy*, 70–77.

7. L. E. Selman et al., "Patients' and Caregivers' Needs, Experiences, Preferences and Research Priorities in Spiritual Care: A Focus Group Study Across Nine Countries," *Palliative Medicine* 32, no. 1 (January 2018), https://doi.org/10.1177/0269216317734954.

8. Jürgen Moltmann, *The Crucified God: The Cross of Christ as the Foundation and Criticism of Christian Theology* (Fortress Press, 1993), 46.

9. Simone Weil, *Waiting on God*, 2nd ed. (Routledge & K. Paul, 1979), 82–83.

10. Michael J. Balboni and Tracy A. Balboni, *Hostility to Hospitality: Spirituality and Professional Socialization within Medicine* (Oxford University Press, 2019), 151–53.

11. We discuss this concept in significant detail in chap. 11 of *Hostility to Hospitality*.

12. *The Rule of Saint Benedict*, chap. 36, https://theruleofbenedict.com/2020/11/13/chapter-36-the-sick/.

Chapter 5 Preparing and Planning

1. Kenneth I. Pargament, *The Psychology of Religion and Coping: Theory, Research, Practice* (Guilford Press, 1997).

2. The first Christian to offer comprehensive remarks about medicine was St. Basil. His remarks concerning Hippocratic medicine can be found in his Long Rules 55 and Short Rules 315. The Long Rules 55 is available for download here: https://www.google.com/url?sa=t&source=web&rct=j&opi=89978449&url=https://cmacincy.org/wp-content/uploads/2020/11/Basils-Long-Rule-Q55-1.docx&ved=2ahUKEwjeg9m0ht-JAxV0GlkFHezuKJsQFnoECBYQAQ&usg=AOvVaw0Tvje8SVHmySvTfqAAXXwT. For a critical print edition, see Anna Silvas, *The Asketikon of St Basil the Great*, Oxford Early Christian Studies (Oxford University Press, 2005).

3. J. E. Pérez and A. Rex Smith, "Intrinsic Religiousness and Well-Being Among Cancer Patients: The Mediating Role of Control-Related Religious Coping and Self-Efficacy for Coping with Cancer," *Journal of Behavioral Medicine* 38, no. 2 (April 2015), https://doi.org/10.1007/s10865-014-9593-2; B. McLaughlin et al., "It Is Out of My Hands: How Deferring Control to God Can Decrease Quality of Life for Breast Cancer Patients," *Psycho-Oncology* 22, no. 12 (December 2013), https://doi.org/10.1002/pon.3356.

4. T. A. Balboni et al., "A Scale to Assess Religious Beliefs in End-of-Life Medical Care," *Cancer* 125, no. 9 (May 1, 2019), https://doi.org/10.1002/cncr.31946.

5. S. R. Alcorn et al., "'If God Wanted Me Yesterday, I Wouldn't Be Here Today': Religious and Spiritual Themes in Patients' Experiences of Advanced Cancer," *Journal of Palliative Medicine* 13, no. 5 (May 2010), https://doi.org/10.1089/jpm.2009.0343.

6. Balboni et al., "Scale to Assess Religious Beliefs in End-of-Life Medical Care."

7. Thomas Aquinas, *Summa Theologica*, II-II q.47 a.1 ad 1.

8. Thomas G. Long, *Accompany Them with Singing: The Christian Funeral* (Westminster John Knox Press, 2009).

9. Medicare pays hospice care by the day depending on the type of care a patient needs. Routine hospice at home gives support through short visits and help from family, while inpatient hospice provides constant and intense nursing care in a medical setting. Using the 2026 rates, home hospice is paid much less each day (about $230) than inpatient hospice (about $1,150 to $1,250) because inpatient care requires staff to always be available. These differences often affect what choices patients have at the end of life.

10. M. J. Balboni et al., "U.S. Clergy Religious Values and Relationships to End-of-Life Discussions and Care," *Journal of Pain and Symptom Management* 53, no. 6 (June 2017), https://doi.org/10.1016/j.jpainsymman.2016.12.346. Of course, larger, urban congregations tend to have clusters of physicians and nurses; whereas many smaller, rural churches may have few, if any, medical professionals.

Chapter 6 Addressing Miracles and Fears

1. Tyler J. VanderWeele, *A Theology of Health: Wholeness and Human Flourishing* (University of Notre Dame Press, 2024), 251.

2. Herman N. Ridderbos, *The Coming of the Kingdom* (P&R, 1962), chap. 3.

3. Michael S. Heiser, *The Unseen Realm: Discovering the Supernatural World of the Bible*, exp. ed. (Lexham Press, 2025).

4. St. Augustine, *The City of God, Books XVII–XXII*, trans. Gerald G. Walsh and Daniel J. Honan, Fathers of the Church: A New Translation 24 (Catholic University of America Press, 1954), book 22, chap. 8, 452.

5. Kate Bowler, *Blessed: A History of the American Prosperity Gospel* (Oxford University Press, 2013), 177.

6. D. P. Sulmasy, "What Is a Miracle?," *Southern Medical Journal* 100, no. 12 (December 2007), https://doi.org/10.1097/SMJ.0b013e31815a9784.

7. Jacalyn Duffin, *Medical Miracles: Doctors, Saints, and Healing in the Modern World* (Oxford University Press, 2009).

8. M. J. Balboni et al., "U.S. Clergy Religious Values and Relationships to End-of-Life Discussions and Care," *Journal of Pain and Symptom Management* 53, no. 6 (June 2017), https://doi.org/10.1016/j.jpainsymman.2016.12.346.

9. R. B. Gaffin, "A Cessationist View," in *Are Miraculous Gifts for Today? 4 Views*, ed. Stanley N. Gundry and Wayne A. Grudem (Zondervan Academic, 1996), 57.

10. Craig S. Keener, *Miracles: The Credibility of the New Testament Accounts*, 2 vols. (Baker Academic, 2011), 2:604–5.

11. "Healing Is the Will of God for You," Kenneth Hagin Ministries, accessed January 15, 2026, https://events.rhema.org/hf-march-4/.

12. Excellent introductions to health care chaplaincy include: Wendy Cadge, *Paging God: Religion in the Halls of Medicine* (University of Chicago Press, 2012); Wendy Cadge and Shelly Rambo, eds., *Chaplaincy and Spiritual Care in the Twenty-First Century: An Introduction* (University of North Carolina Press, 2022); George Fitchett, *Assessing Spiritual Needs: A Guide for Caregivers* (Augsburg Fortress, 2002); George Fitchett, *Spiritual Care in Practice: Case Studies in Healthcare Chaplaincy* (Jessica Kingsley Publishers, 2015).

13. Paul R. Williamson, *Death and the Afterlife: Biblical Perspectives on Ultimate Questions* (InterVarsity, 2018), 54.

14. St. Augustine, *City of God*, 510–11.

Chapter 7 Struggle and Longing

1. Kenneth I. Pargament and Julie J. Exline, *Working with Spiritual Struggles in Psychotherapy: From Research to Practice* (Guilford Press, 2022), 12–15.

2. Pargament and Exline, *Working with Spiritual Struggles*, 14.

3. S. D. W. King et al., "Religious/Spiritual Struggle in Young Adult Hematopoietic Cell Transplant Survivors," *Journal of Adolescent and Young Adult Oncology* 7, no. 2 (April 2018), https://doi.org/10.1089/jayao.2017.0069; R. Hebert et al., "Positive and Negative Religious Coping and Well-Being in Women with Breast Cancer," *Journal of Palliative Medicine* 12, no. 6 (June 2009), https://doi.org/10.1089/jpm.2008.0250; G. Fitchett et al., "Religious Struggle: Prevalence, Correlates and Mental Health Risks in Diabetic, Congestive Heart Failure, and Oncology Patients," *International Journal of Psychiatry in Medicine* 34, no. 2 (2004), https://doi.org/10.2190/UCJ9-DP4M-9C0X-835M.

4. K. E. Steinhauser et al., "Factors Considered Important at the End of Life by Patients, Family, Physicians, and Other Care Providers," *JAMA* 284, no. 19 (November 15, 2000), https://doi.org/10.1001/jama.284.19.2476.

5. A. Damen et al., "Prevalence, Predictors and Correlates of Religious and Spiritual Struggles in Palliative Cancer Patients," *Journal of Pain and Symptom Management* 62, no. 3 (September 2021), https://doi.org/10.1016/j.jpainsymman.2021.04.024.

6. W. D. Winkelman et al., "The Relationship of Spiritual Concerns to the Quality of Life of Advanced Cancer Patients: Preliminary Findings," *Journal of Palliative Medicine* 14, no. 9 (September 2011), https://doi.org/10.1089/jpm.2010.0536.

7. A. B. Astrow et al., "Spiritual Needs and Perception of Quality of Care and Satisfaction with Care in Hematology/Medical Oncology Patients: A Multicultural Assessment," *Journal of Pain and Symptom Management* 55, no. 1 (January 2018): 56–64.

8. We reported her case in Michael J. Balboni and Tracy A. Balboni, *Hostility to Hospitality: Spirituality and Professional Socialization within Medicine* (Oxford University Press, 2019), 31.

9. Viktor E. Frankl, *Man's Search for Meaning* (Beacon Press, 2024).

10. Mark Mather, "The Demography of Dementia and Dementia Caregiving," *Today's Research on Aging*, no. 40 (2020).

11. John Swinton, *Dementia: Living in the Memories of God* (Eerdmans, 2012).

12. Tricia Williams, *What Happens to Faith When Christians Get Dementia? The Faith Experience and Practice of Evangelical Christians Living with Mild to Moderate Dementia* (Pickwick, 2021).

13. Kenneth L. Carder, *Ministry with the Forgotten: Dementia Through a Spiritual Lens* (Abingdon, 2019).

14. Arthur Kleinman, *The Soul of Care: The Moral Education of a Husband and a Doctor* (Viking, 2019).

15. Kleinman, *Soul of Care*, 244.
16. Kleinman, *Soul of Care*, 170.

Chapter 8 Seeking Life, Accepting Death

1. T. A. Balboni et al., "A Scale to Assess Religious Beliefs in End-of-Life Medical Care," *Cancer* 125, no. 9 (May 1, 2019), https://doi.org/10.1002/cncr.31946.

2. M. R. Keene et al., "Complementary and Alternative Medicine Use in Cancer: A Systematic Review," *Complementary Therapies in Clinical Practice* 35 (May 2019), https://doi.org/10.1016/j.ctcp.2019.01.004.

3. Complementary and alternative therapies can serve patients well when they are used alongside medical treatment to ease symptoms, reduce suffering, and support emotional and psychological well-being. Practices with strong evidence (e.g., mind-body and movement-based therapies) may offer real comfort, reducing anxiety and depression and enhancing quality of life as patients face serious illness. At the same time, wisdom and caution are needed when evidence is limited and promises grow large, especially when hope is tied to treatments that claim more than they can deliver or pull patients away from proven care. See L. E. Carlson et al., "Integrative Oncology Care of Symptoms of Anxiety and Depression in Adults with Cancer: Society for Integrative Oncology-ASCO Guideline," *Journal of Clinical Oncology* 41, no. 28 (October 1, 2023), https://doi.org/10.1200/jco.23.00857.

4. Balboni et al., "Scale to Assess Religious Beliefs"; M. J. Balboni et al., "U.S. Clergy Religious Values and Relationships to End-of-Life Discussions and Care," *Journal of Pain and Symptom Management* 53, no. 6 (June 2017), https://doi.org/10.1016/j.jpainsymman.2016.12.346.

5. Balboni et al., "U.S. Clergy Religious Values."

6. Allen Verhey, *The Christian Art of Dying: Learning from Jesus* (Eerdmans, 2011), 154.

7. Verhey, *Christian Art of Dying*, 154.

8. Verhey, *Christian Art of Dying*, 154.

9. J. J. Sanders et al., "Seeking and Accepting: U.S. Clergy Theological and Moral Perspectives Informing Decision Making at the End of Life," *Journal of Palliative Medicine* 20, no. 10 (October 2017), https://doi.org/10.1089/jpm.2016.0545.

10. "Respect for Human Life," Catechism of the Catholic Church (Libreria Editrice Vaticana, 1993), 3.2.2.5.1:2278–79, https://www.vatican.va/archive/ENG0015/__P7Z.HTM.

11. Winston T. Smith, "Hospital Visitation: Become a Companion in the Wilderness," *Journal of Biblical Counseling* 29, no. 3 (2015): 8–20.

Chapter 9 Forgiveness

1. T. S. Eliot, "Burnt Norton," *Four Quartets*, in *The Complete Poems and Plays 1909–1950* (Harcourt Brace & Company, 1950), 111.

2. B. Ferrell et al., "Nurses' Responses to Requests for Forgiveness at the End of Life," *Journal of Pain and Symptom Management* 47, no. 3 (March 2014), https://doi.org/10.1016/j.jpainsymman.2013.05.009.

3. M. Ratshikana-Moloko et al., "Spiritual Care, Pain Reduction, and Preferred Place of Death Among Advanced Cancer Patients in Soweto, South Africa," *Journal of Pain and Symptom Management* 60, no. 1 (July 2020), https://doi.org/10.1016/j.jpainsymman.2020.01.019.

4. K. N. G. Long et al., "Forgiveness of Others and Subsequent Health and Well-being in Mid-Life: A Longitudinal Study on Female Nurses," *BMC Psychology* 8, no. 1 (October 1, 2020), https://doi.org/10.1186/s40359-020-00470-w.

5. J. Kim, J. Hulett, and S. P. Heiney, "Forgiveness and Health Outcomes in Cancer Survivorship: A Scoping Review," *Cancer Nursing* 44, no. 4 (July–August 2021), https://doi.org/10.1097/ncc.0000000000000809.

6. L. L. Toussaint et al., "The Relationship Between Forgiveness and Health Outcomes Among People Living with HIV: A Cross-Sectional Study in France," *AIDS and Behavior* 27, no. 10 (October 2023), https://doi.org/10.1007/s10461-023-04052-w.

7. R. S. Silva et al., "Forgiveness Facilitation in Palliative Care: A Scoping Review," *JBI Evidence Synthesis* 18, no. 11 (November 2020), https://doi.org/10.11124/jbisrir-d-19-00286.

8. Everett L. Worthington, *Five Steps to Forgiveness: The Art and Science of Forgiving* (Crown, 2001); Everett L. Worthington, *Forgiveness and Reconciliation: Theory and Application* (Routledge, 2006); Everett L. Worthington, *A Just Forgiveness: Responsible Healing Without Excusing Injustice* (InterVarsity, 2009).

9. Everett L. Worthington, *Moving Forward: Six Steps to Forgiving Yourself and Breaking Free from the Past* (WaterBrook, 2013).

10. T. J. VanderWeele, "Is Forgiveness a Public Health Issue?," *American Journal of Public Health* 108, no. 2 (February 2018), https://doi.org/10.2105/ajph.2017.304210; Worthington, *A Just Forgiveness*.

11. S. R. Alcorn et al., "'If God Wanted Me Yesterday, I Wouldn't Be Here Today': Religious and Spiritual Themes in Patients' Experiences of Advanced Cancer," *Journal of Palliative Medicine* 13, no. 5 (May 2010), https://doi.org/10.1089/jpm.2009.0343.

12. Kim, Hulett, and Heiney, "Forgiveness and Health Outcomes."

13. M. Renz et al., "Forgiveness and Reconciliation Processes in Dying Patients with Cancer," *American Journal of Hospice and Palliative Medicine* 37, no. 3 (March 2020), https://doi.org/10.1177/1049909119867675.

14. Worthington, *Forgiveness and Reconciliation*.

15. E. L. Worthington Jr., adapted from Richard Cowden and Kate Jackson-Meyer, *Reach Forgiveness Workbook, Adapted for Churches* (2025). For this and other resources, visit Harvard's Human Flourishing Program at hfh.fas.harvard.edu/forgiveness.

Chapter 10 Medicine, Pain, and Hope

1. See Michael J. Balboni and Tracy A. Balboni, *Hostility to Hospitality: Spirituality and Professional Socialization Within Medicine* (Oxford University Press, 2019), chap. 12.

2. Basil of Caesarea, *Saint Basil: Ascetical Works*, trans. M. Monica Wagner (Catholic University of America Press, 1962), 336.

3. Balboni and Balboni, *Hostility to Hospitality*, chap. 10.

4. Dr. Christina Puchalski's spiritual care training program at the George Washington University School of Medicine and Health Sciences offers brief opportunities for clinicians of all faiths or none to learn how to navigate matters of spirituality in patient care. For more information, visit the GW Institute for Spirituality and Health website: https://gwish.smhs.gwu.edu.

5. Francis R. Packard, *The Life and Times of Ambroise Paré (1510–1590)* (Paul B. Hoeber, 1921), 160.

6. We especially recommend the Christian Medical and Dental Association (www.CMDA.org), the International Christian Medical and Dental Association (www.ICMDA.net), and the Catholic Medical Association (www.cathmed.org). For theological training at this intersection, Duke Divinity School's Theology, Medicine, and Culture Program is exceptional (https://divinity.duke.edu/initiatives/tmc).

7. David Clark, "'Total Pain': Disciplinary Power and the Body in the Work of Cicely Saunders, 1958–1967," *Social Science & Medicine* 49, no. 6 (1999): 727–36.

8. T. A. Balboni et al., "A Scale to Assess Religious Beliefs in End-of-Life Medical Care," *Cancer* 125, no. 9 (May 1, 2019), https://doi.org/10.1002/cncr.31946.

9. J. J. Sanders et al., "Seeking and Accepting: U.S. Clergy Theological and Moral Perspectives Informing Decision Making at the End of Life," *Journal of Palliative Medicine* 20, no. 10 (October 2017), https://doi.org/10.1089/jpm.2016.0545.

10. W. D. Winkelman et al., "The Relationship of Spiritual Concerns to the Quality of Life of Advanced Cancer Patients: Preliminary Findings," *Journal of Palliative Medicine* 14, no. 9 (September 2011), https://doi.org/10.1089/jpm.2010.0536.

11. A. Damen et al., "Prevalence, Predictors and Correlates of Religious and Spiritual Struggles in Palliative Cancer Patients," *Journal of Pain and Symptom Management* 62, no. 3 (September 2021), https://doi.org/10.1016/j.jpainsymman.2021.04.024.

12. Kai A. D. Morgan et al., "Associations Amongst Disease Severity, Religious Coping and Depression in a Cohort of Jamaicans with Sickle-Cell Disease," *Mental Health, Religion & Culture* 17, no. 9 (2014), https://doi.org/10.1080/13674676.2014.961910.

13. J. J. Exline and J. A. Wilt, "Supernatural Attributions: Seeing God, the Devil, Demons, Spirits, Fate, and Karma as Causes of Events," *Annual Review of Clinical Psychology* 19 (May 9, 2023), https://doi.org/10.1146/annurev-clinpsy-080921-081114.

14. Kate Bowler, *Everything Happens for a Reason: And Other Lies I've Loved* (Random House, 2018), 116–22.

15. Julian of Norwich, *Revelations of Divine Love*, trans. Barry Windeatt (Oxford University Press, 2015), 20.

Chapter 11 Circle of Love

1. T. A. Balboni et al., "Religiousness and Spiritual Support Among Advanced Cancer Patients and Associations with End-of-Life Treatment Preferences and Quality of Life," *Journal of Clinical Oncology* 25, no. 5 (February 10, 2007), https://doi.org/10.1200/JCO.2006.07.9046.

2. Guenter B. Risse, *Mending Bodies, Saving Souls: A History of Hospitals* (Oxford University Press, 1999), 105.

3. See Susan J. Dunlap, *Caring Cultures: How Congregations Respond to the Sick* (Baylor University Press, 2009).

4. Dunlap, *Caring Cultures*, chaps. 1–2.

5. M. J. Balboni et al., "Why Is Spiritual Care Infrequent at the End of Life? Spiritual Care Perceptions Among Patients, Nurses, and Physicians and the Role of Training," *Journal of Clinical Oncology* 31, no. 4 (February 1, 2013), https://doi.org/10.1200/JCO.2012.44.6443.

6. Thomas C. Oden, *Pastoral Theology: Essentials of Ministry* (Harper & Row, 1982), 101.

7. Karen Lampe, *The Caring Congregation Ministry: Care Minister's Manual* (Abingdon, 2021).

8. V. T. LeBaron et al., "How Community Clergy Provide Spiritual Care: Toward a Conceptual Framework for Clergy End-of-Life Education," *Journal of Pain and Symptom Management* 51, no. 4 (April 2016), https://doi.org/10.1016/j.jpainsymman.2015.11.016.

9. M. J. Balboni et al., "U.S. Clergy Religious Values and Relationships to End-of-Life Discussions and Care," *Journal of Pain and Symptom Management* 53, no. 6 (June 2017), https://doi.org/10.1016/j.jpainsymman.2016.12.346.

10. See Here to Honor (https://heretohonor.com), The Conversation Project (https://theconversationproject.org/faith/), and Five Wishes (https://www.fivewishes.org).

11. Kathryn Butler, *Between Life and Death: A Gospel-Centered Guide to End-of-Life Medical Care* (Crossway, 2019).

Chapter 12 A Community of Presence

1. Readers can explore this concept in pastoral care writings such as John Patton, *Pastoral Care in Context: An Introduction to Pastoral Care* (Westminster John Knox, 1993); William A. Clebsch and Charles R. Jaekle, *Pastoral Care in Historical Perspective* (Jason Aronson, 1983); Carrie Doehring, *The Practice of Pastoral Care: A Postmodern Approach* (Westminster John Knox, 2006).

2. One book that illustrates this point in detail is Kate Bowler, *Everything Happens for a Reason: And Other Lies I've Loved* (Random House, 2018).

Chapter 13 Dancing with Lois

1. GriefShare is a thirteen-week support group for those grieving the loss of a loved one. It has a Christian foundation but is intentionally broad to welcome all. See https://www.griefshare.org.

2. V. T. LeBaron et al., "Clergy Views on a Good Versus a Poor Death: Ministry to the Terminally Ill," *Journal of Palliative Medicine* 18, no. 12 (December 2015), https://doi.org/10.1089/jpm.2015.0176.

3. "Physician assisted suicide," also called by advocates "physician aid in dying," refers to situations in which patients who doctors say cannot be cured and are likely to die within six months request from their physician medication intended to cause death, which the patient must take on their own. "Euthanasia"

refers to a practice in which a physician directly administers medication intended to cause death. In the United States, physician assisted suicide is limited to consenting adults with a terminal prognosis of less than six months. As of 2026, thirteen states have legalized PAS. In Canada and several European countries where euthanasia is legal, eligibility can include adults or, in some places, minors with a grievous and irremediable medical condition, which can include certain mental health disorders.

4. M. J. Balboni et al., "The Views of Clergy Regarding Ethical Controversies in Care at the End of Life," *Journal of Pain and Symptom Management* 55, no. 1 (January 2018), https://doi.org/10.1016/j.jpainsymman.2017.05.009.

5. D. P. Sulmasy et al., "Non-Faith-Based Arguments Against Physician-Assisted Suicide and Euthanasia," *Linacre Quarterly* 83, no. 3 (August 2016), https://doi.org/10.1080/00243639.2016.1201375; Kathleen M. Foley and Herbert Hendin, *The Case Against Assisted Suicide: For the Right to End-of-Life Care* (Johns Hopkins University Press, 2002).

6. Farr A. Curlin and Christopher Tollefsen, *The Way of Medicine: Ethics and the Healing Profession*, Notre Dame studies in Medical Ethics and Bioethics (University of Notre Dame Press, 2021).

7. Thomas C. Oden, *Life in the Spirit*, vol. 3 of *Systematic Theology* (Harper SanFrancisco, 1992), 392–97.

8. C. S. Lewis, *The Great Divorce: A Dream* (HarperSanFrancisco, 2001), 75.

9. Lewis, *The Great Divorce*, 75.

10. Thomas G. Long, *Accompany Them with Singing: The Christian Funeral* (Westminster John Knox, 2009).

11. Congregation for the Doctrine of the Faith, *Instruction Ad resurgendum cum Christo Regarding the Burial of the Deceased and the Conservation of the Ashes in the Case of Cremation*, The Holy See, 2016, https://www.vatican.va/roman_curia/congregations/cfaith/documents/rc_con_cfaith_doc_20160815_ad-resurgendum-cum-christo_en.html.

12. Jean Calvin, *Institutes of the Christian Religion*, vol. 2, The Library of Christian Classics (Westminster, 1960), 882–83.

13. Dennis Klass, Phyllis R. Silverman, and Steven L. Nickman, *Continuing Bonds: New Understandings of Grief* (Taylor & Francis, 1996).

14. Robert A. Neimeyer, *Meaning Reconstruction and the Experience of Loss* (American Psychological Association, 2001); Melissa M. Kelley, *Grief: Contemporary Theory and the Practice of Ministry* (Fortress, 2010).

15. Mark Vroegop, *Dark Clouds, Deep Mercy: Discovering the Grace of Lament* (Crossway, 2019).

16. J. A. Groves, "Nourishing Your Emotional Life," *Journal of Biblical Counseling* 32, no. 1 (2018): 48–62.

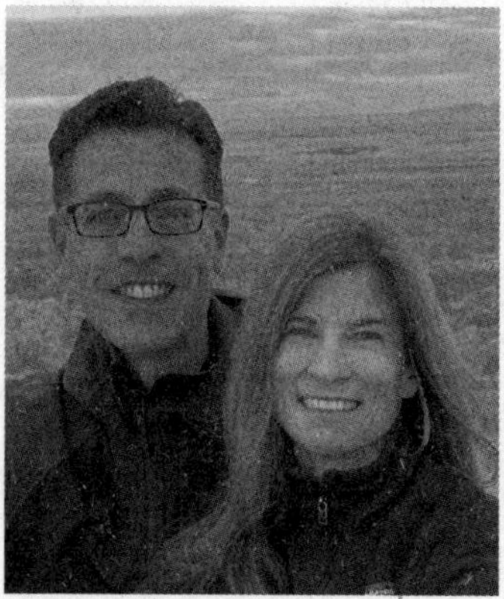

About the Authors

Tracy Balboni, MD, and **Michael Balboni**, PhD, a wife-and-husband team, serve as researchers, professional caregivers, and codirectors of the Harvard Initiative on Health, Spirituality, and Religion. Tracy is a professor at Harvard Medical School, an internationally known researcher in palliative care, and director of the Harvard Radiation Oncology residency program. Michael is a theologian and scholar on spirituality and medicine at Harvard and serves as a pastor at Restoration Fellowship and the Longwood Christian Community, both in Boston, Massachusetts.

Connect with
Michael and Tracy at
WalkingLoisHome.com.